NATURE AND NURTURE IN PSYCHIATRY

A Predisposition–Stress Model of Mental Disorders

NATURE AND NURTURE IN PSYCHIATRY

*A Predisposition–Stress Model
of Mental Disorders*

By

Joel Paris, M.D.

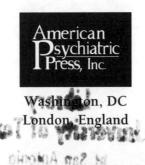

American Psychiatric Press, Inc.

Washington, DC
London, England

Copyright © 1999 American Psychiatric Press, Inc.
ALL RIGHTS RESERVED
Manufactured in the United States of America on acid-free paper
02 01 00 99   4 3 2 1
First Edition

American Psychiatric Press, Inc.
1400 K Street, N.W., Washington, DC   20005
www.appi.org

Library of Congress Cataloging-in-Publication Data
Paris, Joel, 1940-.
    Nature and nurture in psychiatry : a predisposition-stress model of mental disorders / by Joel Paris. — 1st ed.
        p.   cm.
    Includes bibliographical references and index.
    ISBN 0-88048-781-X
    1.   Mental illness—Genetic aspects.   2.   Stress (Psychology).
3.   Psychology, Pathological.   I.   Title.
    [DNLM: 1.   Mental Disorders—genetics.   2.   Mental Disorders—psychology.   3.   Stress, Psychological.   4.   Models, Psychological.   WM 140P232n 1998]
   RC455.4.G4P37   1998
   616.89'042—dc21
   DNLM/DLC   98-26811
   for Library of Congress   CIP

British Library Cataloguing in Publication Data
A CIP record is available from the British Library.

This book is dedicated to
Sir Michael Rutter.

Contents

PART III: IMPLICATIONS

Introduction

Nature and Nurture

Humanity is a single species. All of us have a great deal in common. We share the same body plan. We also have similar patterns of thought.

Yet we are very different from each other. Humans differ in physical characteristics, such as height, facial features, and skin color. We are also mentally different—in our thoughts, in our emotions, and in our behavior.

What is the source of this variability among individuals? Physical differences have always been understood as being related to genetic factors. However, mental differences have not always been seen in the same way. Over the centuries, philosophers and scientists have addressed the *nature–nurture* dilemma—Are we mainly a product of our genes, or are we largely a product of our environment?

This issue has been the center of intense controversy in psychiatry. For example, clinicians and researchers continue to debate whether clinical depression derives from a "chemical imbalance" or is usually a response to loss and disappointment. Similar debates have raged over the origins of other mental disorders.

This book will address the question of the *relative* importance of nature and nurture in psychiatric disorders. It will do so not through polemics, but rather through a careful examination of empirical evidence. Not surprisingly, in most cases, the debate can only be resolved by recognizing the importance of *both* nature and nurture. However, when the answer to a question is "all of the above," we run the risk of oversimplifying the problem. We need to know how genes and environment *interact* with each other to produce mental disorders. We also need to understand the mechanisms of these interactions.

■ The Origins of This Book

This book has both intellectual and personal roots. One of my motivations in writing it was to summarize what I have learned in 30 years as a psychiatrist. At the same time, I want to share with readers what I have had to *unlearn*.

When I began my training in the 1960s, like many North American residents during that time, I was taught that the causes of most common mental disorders in adults lie, for the most part, in an unhappy childhood. Psychodynamic models framed the understanding of nearly every form of psychopathology. Even though these ideas were inaccurate, they were intellectually exciting and seductive.

When I began to practice psychiatry, I identified with my teachers and worked within a similar framework. Since I was interested in the long-term treatment of personality disorders, and since most of my patients were young adults suitable for psychotherapy, a psychodynamic model seemed to have the most to offer.

Like most clinicians, I started with high hopes but achieved mixed success. Some patients did brilliantly—these are the cases clinicians like to write up! Other patients deteriorated despite my best efforts. Most patients showed middling levels of improvement.

As a teacher of psychiatric residents, I also took a strongly psychodynamic perspective. Whatever the presenting problems, I could come up with a plausible explanation for them based on the details of the patient's personal history. Recently, I have thought that I should undertake a "product recall" and inform my residents from the early 1970s to ignore my earlier approaches to formulation. However, since my former students have already forgotten most of what I taught them, this warning is probably unnecessary!

In the course of my career, my ideas about psychiatry have changed dramatically. Over the last 25 years I have run an outpatient clinic that evaluates large numbers of new patients. I have now seen about 10,000 patients—approximately the population of a small town. Exposure to a broad range of pathology has helped me to appreciate the complexity of the pathways to mental illness.

I have also been fortunate to have colleagues who helped me, at midcareer, to develop a second career as a clinical researcher. In spite of my late arrival on the scientific scene, there were some advantages to having begun as a clinician–teacher. My experiences as a therapist led me to address questions as to why some patients, under stressful circumstances, develop one type of illness, while other patients, faced with the same stressors, develop a completely different type of illness.

In my research, I focused on patients with personality disorders, a group that all too often fails to benefit from psychotherapy. Traditionally, clinicians believed that the intractability of personality problems derived from their roots in early childhood. However, I have concluded that life events alone cannot account for the development of personality disorders—or, for that matter, of most mental disorders.

Four lines of evidence support this conclusion:

1. Children who have experienced serious adversity demonstrate high levels of resilience, and many develop no discernible psychopathology.
2. A large number of patients with mental disorders have no history of childhood adversity.
3. Siblings exposed to the same parental environment have different personalities, and, if they should later develop mental disorders, do not necessarily develop the same ones.
4. Patients with similar life experiences can develop completely different illnesses.

When the events in an individual's life have been stressful, it is at least plausible to account for his or her present difficulties by personal history. However, what clinicians do not always realize is that their patients are a highly selected subsample of those who have been exposed to any given stressor. As we will see in the course of this book, when researchers go out into the community and interview nonclinical samples, most people who have been exposed to negative life events have either mild difficulties or none at all.

These facts are very striking indeed. To explain them, we need a better theoretical model. Environmental factors do not account for these discrepancies between personal histories and psychopathology. The answer lies in predisposing factors particular to the individual.

I have addressed these questions in two previous books, one on borderline personality disorder (Paris 1994) and another on all of the personality disorders (Paris 1996a). In both books, I underlined the absence of a clear-cut causal relationship between childhood experiences and adult personality or psychopathology, and suggested that personality disorders arise from interactions between biological predispositions and environmental stressors. The present book expands these ideas into a *general* model that can be applied to most categories of mental disorder.

Beyond Reductionism

The pathways leading to mental disorders are not linear; rather, they involve an enormously complex set of interactions. The principle that disorders have multiple causes is a truism. Yet contemporary psychiatry honors it "more in the breach than in the observance." Like other disciplines, psychiatry has been susceptible to reductionistic theories. Complexity is difficult to grasp. We are tempted to reduce cognitive dissonance and to look for simple ways to explain what we see.

Psychiatry has also suffered from what Snow (1958/1993) called the problem of "two cultures"—that is, a division between the point of view of science and that of the humanities. Thus, one psychiatric culture is strongly biomedical (Kirmayer 1994b). Its world view is that mental disorders are primarily the result of factors *within* the person, most particularly physiological and/or biochemical abnormalities. The second culture is psychosocial and environmental. Its world view is that mental disorders primarily result from factors *outside* the person. Yet both these views are *reductionistic* and are based on unidimensional theories.

Biological reductionism dominated psychiatry in the 19th century but went into relative decline in the first half of the 20th century. Today, in this "decade of the brain," biology has again come to dominate psychiatric theory. Unfortunately, contemporary neurobiological models oversimplify the role of genetic factors and often fail to address the role of the psychosocial precipitating factors that determine whether mental disorders emerge from underlying predispositions.

Environmental reductionism in psychiatry reached the peak of its influence during the 1950s and 1960s and then went into a decline. However, this point of view still retains a large constituency among committed psychotherapists. Environmental theories are reductionistic when they oversimplify the role of stressors in psychopathology, assume that single events can cause disorders, and fail to address how stressors interact with underlying diatheses.

The theoretical models we use are not just a matter of intellectual interest. They profoundly affect what we do clinically. When we believe that mental disorders arise from single causes, we tend to treat them with single methods. Thus, if we take a purely biomedical view, we will search for aberrant enzymatic pathways that can be specifically targeted by carefully designed pharmacological agents. Alternatively, if we take a purely environmental view, we will search for life events that can be addressed through psychotherapy.

I will argue in this book that to do justice to the causes of psychopathology, we need much more sophisticated explanations of the relationship between risks and disorders. A comprehensive and clinically relevant approach must be nonreductionistic. Only a complex theory can address the complex origins of psychopathology. This book will aim to demonstrate that an *interactive* model is the best way to understand the causes of mental disorders.

■ The Predisposition–Stress Model

Predisposition–stress theory is a model that has been used widely in medicine. Whenever we apply a "medical model" to psychiatry (Guze 1992), we normally take both predispositions and stressors into account. Psychiatrists of my generation had, of course, been taught that schizophrenia and bipolar illness do not develop without some form of biological vulnerability. What we had not been taught is that virtually *all* forms of psychopathology depend on predispositions. This principle had been taken for granted in the time of Kraepelin, but was largely forgotten in the heyday of psychodynamic psychiatry. On the basis of new genetic evidence, predispositions are returning to the forefront of contemporary theory.

In this model, the impact of life events cannot be understood without considering innate diatheses, and the impact of constitutional vulnerability cannot be understood without considering stressors. (Although, in principle, diatheses and stressors can be either biological or psychosocial, the term *predisposition* usually refers to constitutional factors, while the term *stress* generally refers to psychosocial adversities.)

The predisposition–stress (or stress–diathesis) model has a long and distinguished history in psychiatry (Monroe and Simons 1991). The most influential advocate of this approach in our century was the Swiss–American psychiatrist Adolf Meyer (Muncie 1939). Engel's (1980) "biopsychosocial model" revived and modernized the principles of Meyerian psychiatry, hypothesizing that mental disorders emerge from interactions between biological, psychological, and social factors.

The biopsychosocial model has been helpful in encouraging psychiatrists to think multidimensionally. However, it has one serious defect: it fails to explain why some individuals develop one category of mental disorder while other individuals develop a completely different category of illness. This question can only be addressed by assuming that individual differences in susceptibility to mental disorders are rooted in biological vulnerability.

The predisposition–stress model also provides a way of understanding the interactions between genes and environment. To conceptualize these relationships, it is helpful to emphasize the difference between necessary and sufficient conditions for developing psychopathology. *Necessary* conditions are those without which a mental disorder cannot develop. Predispositions usually constitute the most important necessary conditions for most human diseases. *Sufficient* conditions are those in whose presence a disorder will inevitably develop. These usually consist of the interactive and cumulative effects of both predispositions and stressors. We do not know the sufficient causes of most diseases in medicine. (Highly infectious viral illnesses are obvious exceptions.) Since most diseases have multiple causes, only a complex combination of necessary factors can ever be "sufficient."

Predispositions are usually necessary causes for mental disorders, while stressors are much less specific. Therefore, predispositions have a *privileged* etiological role. Unless a specific vulnerability is present, individuals either will not fall ill or will develop some other form of illness. Moreover, in most cases, no single stressor causes disease. Instead, many stressors are involved, each of which contributes to a cumulative effect. At some point, all of these effects cross a "threshold of liability," producing overt pathology (Falconer 1989).

The model has many interesting implications. One is that the relationship between risks and disorders is *nonlinear*. In other words, risk factors do not by themselves produce pathology, but rather have different effects in vulnerable individuals, in whom a small amount of stress can precipitate severe illness. Clinicians often make the mistake of seeing these precipitating factors as ultimate causes of illness in patients.

Another implication of the model is that similar clinical outcomes can emerge from different etiological pathways. Thus, some patients with a disorder will have stronger predispositions, leading them to become ill at low levels of exposure to stress. Other patients with the same disorder will have weaker predispositions, and will become ill only when exposed to high levels of stress. However, as we will see later in the book, illnesses often show differences in course or symptomatology that depend on the strength of predispositions.

The predisposition–stress model also helps to account for the role of environmental factors in human illness. Predispositions to psychiatric illness vary in their intensity, which explains why the same life events can lead to different outcomes in different individuals. Predispositions determine the thresholds for developing specific psychiatric disorders, and also shape a wider spectrum of outcomes, ranging from overt illness to differences in personality (Meehl 1990).

Predispositions to mental disorders can be measured as *traits*. The relationship between traits and disorders is a crucial aspect of the predisposition–stress model. Individuals may carry genetically determined traits without ever developing any of the disorders associated with them. Thus, for every person who falls ill, there will be many others who have the same trait yet remain well. In many forms of mental illness, the environment is the primary determinant of whether an individual crosses the threshold of liability between trait and disorder.

Let us now consider, as an illustration of the predisposition–stress model, the etiology of tuberculosis. This may not be the first example that most of us would think of, but it is an instructive one. Although infectious diseases cannot develop without the presence of a specific organism, many individuals who have the bacterium causing tuberculosis in their lungs never develop any illness. Therefore, the infectious agent is a necessary but not a sufficient cause of disease. Many other factors—most particularly, genetic predispositions to infection, nutrition, intercurrent disease, as well as immunological factors—determine whether illness will develop (Childs et al. 1992). Tuberculosis becomes clinically apparent only when the cumulative effects of all of these risks cross a threshold.

At the interface between psychiatry and medicine, we can apply the same model to "psychosomatic" disorders. At one time, it was thought that each of these diseases was associated with specific psychodynamic constellations (Alexander 1950). However, empirical research failed to support these conjectures, and most theorists have concluded that whether or not one develops overt pathology depends on stressors, whereas the particular illness that develops is accounted for by predispositions (Weiner 1977).

Finally, we can apply this model to the interface between psychiatry and psychology. A relatively new field of research called *developmental psychopathology* has become an important source of supporting evidence for predisposition–stress theory (Cohler et al. 1995). It is now well established that although negative psychosocial factors increase the risk for many forms of adult mental illness, most children exposed to psychosocial adversities never develop *any* mental disorder (Rutter 1987a; Rutter and Maughan 1997). Children raised by parents with mental disorders, or children with severe psychosocial disadvantages, are *statistically* more likely to become dysfunctional. Yet, in the majority of cases, they become surprisingly well-functioning adults.

Predisposition–stress theory helps to account for all of these observations. Since individuals vary a great deal in their vulnerability to stress, not everyone is affected in the same way. Moreover, psychosocial risk factors are balanced by protective factors that promote resilience. On the one hand, every additional negative psychological experience increases the overall risk, leading to cumulative effects that can eventually cross the threshold of liability. On the other hand, every positive experience can reduce the overall risk, lowering the threshold of liability.

The fact that most children at high risk fail to develop mental illness is described by an important construct termed *resilience* (Rutter 1987a). In the presence of environmental risk factors for psychopathology, protective factors in development help most individuals to develop normally. Some of these are biological, such as favorable personality traits. Others derive from fortunate environmental circumstances. Resilience allows children to surmount the most severe disadvantages. The same principle also applies to adversities in adulthood. As we will see later in this book, research has consistently shown that even the most stressful experiences in adult life cause psychopathology only in a minority of cases.

These conclusions do not imply in any way that the psychosocial risk factors for psychiatric illness are unimportant. Rather, what the evidence suggests is that we must be cautious in attributing the pathology of patients *only* to negative events in their lives. Clinicians, because they see only patients who are overtly disordered, tend to develop a distorted view of the relationship between adversity and illness. Negative events have a stronger effect on individuals who are biologically vulnerable. Thus, unless they activate predispositions, even the most severe experiences usually cause only short-term, not long-term, effects (Yehuda and McFarlane 1995).

The general principle is that *most people exposed to stressful events do not develop psychopathology*. It follows that most of the associations in the literature between psychosocial risks and mental disorders are accounted for by predisposed subpopulations.

In summary, the predisposition–stress model represents a major improvement over the simpler theories that previously dominated psychiatry. Thinking interactively helps us to avoid assuming simple relationships between causes and effects. Instead, the model encourages us to address complex relationships between many causes and many effects. It offers a nonreductionistic way of conceptualizing the origins of psychopathology.

Most contemporary clinicians subscribe, at least in principle, to predisposition–stress theory. However, they often only pay it lip service, easily relapsing into linear thinking. Unfortunately, reductionism remains alive and well in psychiatric practice! Clinicians of the future will need to become comfortable with complexity. In the long run, the weight of scientific evidence will change the way we think about mental illness.

■ The Purpose of This Book

This volume does not aim to present a new or an *original* theory of mental disorders. I am hardly the first author to advocate a predisposition–stress model! On the contrary, many others have taken the same point of view, and the theory corresponds to the mainstream position of contemporary psychiatry. The idea that diseases arise from interactions between constitution and experience can be traced as far back as the writings of

Galen (Monroe and Simons 1991). Although many authors have contributed to the model in the last few decades, particular tribute is due to the eloquent and persuasive writings of Herbert Weiner (1977), Gordon Claridge (1985), Michael Rutter (1991), and Goldberg and Huxley (1992).

In addition, a few words are needed to explain what this book will *not* be about. There has been a great deal of research concerning the precise mechanisms that mediate biological predispositions to mental illness. Yet despite all the progress made in recent years, we are still very far from defining how genes act on brain chemistry. Therefore, although this is one of the "hottest" areas of research in psychiatry, this volume will deal with neurobiological mechanisms only peripherally. One can study gene–environment interactions without knowing exactly *how* they affect neurotransmitters, receptors, or chemical messengers. Moreover, this is a fast-changing field, in which today's breakthrough often becomes tomorrow's blind alley. In the future, when these issues are better understood, we will be in a position to develop a predisposition–stress model fully grounded in neurobiology.

In summary, the purpose of this book is to provide the reader with a clear and intelligible summary of the predisposition–stress model and to illustrate its application to the understanding of mental disorders. In showing how the model can be usefully applied to a very wide range of psychopathology, I have had to review an extensive literature indeed. This has involved making compromises between the needs of different readers. Specialists may find some of the discussion lacking in detail concerning either methodology or mechanism. However, this book is primarily aimed at practicing clinicians.

In science, difficult problems are rarely settled by single studies. Only the overall weight of evidence allows reasonably firm conclusions. This is why I have referenced many of my conclusions with review articles or books, which are themselves summaries of the research literature. However, where individual papers shed particular light on questions, I have highlighted these sources. In fact, most of the references in this book consist of research reports published in scientific journals. It is, nevertheless, impossible to review a complex literature without picking and choosing. Wherever my conclusions seem controversial, readers should pursue their own inquiries, making use of the extensive reference list provided at the end of this book.

▇ The Argument of the Chapters

Chapter 1 reviews the historical background of the nature–nurture debate in psychiatry. Over time, the orientation of the discipline has swung back and forth. However, favoring nature or nurture as a cause of mental disorders has usually made a difference in how practitioners treat their patients.

Chapter 2 offers an overview of the mechanisms by which genes shape the predispositions to medical and psychiatric illnesses. In this chapter I demonstrate how individual variations in susceptibility are measured: through twin studies, adoption studies, family history studies, biological markers, and genetic mapping. The underlying continuity between health and disease leads to the conclusion that the genetic mechanisms behind illness can best be understood by means of a *threshold* model.

Chapter 3 presents an overview of the mechanisms by which environmental stressors precipitate mental disorders. In this chapter I offer a critique of the commonly held idea that early childhood experience is the determining factor in adult psychopathology. The range of life stressors involved in psychopathology are reviewed, and the importance of social factors in psychiatric illness is underlined. Finally, I explore the ways in which gene–environment interactions influence both the presence and the impact of stressful life events.

Chapter 4 describes the role of nature and nurture in psychoanalytic theory. Psychoanalysis, although not originally an environmentalist model, has come to be associated with the idea of the primacy of early experience as well as the assumption that childhood determines both adult personality and adult psychopathology. In this chapter I suggest ways in which psychoanalytic theory might be modified to take the role of predispositions into account.

Chapter 5 examines the nature–nurture problem in the social sciences. These disciplines aim to understand normal human behavior and have addressed issues similar to those facing psychiatry. Until recently, environmental models dominated social science theory. In this chapter I examine a few of the controversies that have led psychologists, sociologists, and anthropologists to challenge that point of view.

Chapter 6 demonstrates how a predisposition–stress model accounts for the etiology of many chronic medical illnesses. In it I consider several diseases in which stressors act to uncover underlying vulnerabilities. Coronary artery disease is discussed in some detail, augmented with capsule reviews of research on other common illnesses.

Chapter 7 addresses the problems in defining relationships among disorders, diagnoses, and traits. In this chapter I discuss the boundaries of mental disorders, the criteria used to validate diagnoses in psychiatry, and the concept that mental disorders are maladaptive versions of adaptive traits.

The next eight chapters demonstrate the application of the predisposition–stress model to the major disorders in psychiatry. Each of these chapters is structured in the same way: 1) reviews of evidence for heritability, 2) reviews of evidence for the role of environmental stressors, and 3) models of gene–environment interaction.

Chapter 8 applies the predisposition–stress model to schizophrenia, a disorder that has been a historical battleground between biological and environmental reductionism. Although schizophrenia is now known to have a primarily biological basis, it nicely exemplifies the interactions between predispositions and stressors.

Chapter 9 focuses on mood disorders, a highly heterogeneous group: in bipolar illness, predispositions are primary etiological factors; in severe unipolar depression, predispositions are also crucially important; and in milder unipolar depression, stressors play a more important role.

Chapter 10 examines anxiety disorders. Both predispositions and stressors play a role in panic, phobia, and obsessive-compulsive disorders. In this chapter I also briefly review the etiology of other diagnoses previously classified as "neuroses": somatization and conversion disorders.

Chapter 11 addresses posttraumatic stress disorder. Traumatic theories of psychopathology have often been used to support environmental reductionism. However, research actually shows that traumatic events rarely lead to predictable long-term effects. While the short-term sequelae of traumatic events are determined by the nature of the trauma itself, long-term effects often depend on predispositions.

Chapter 12 examines substance use disorders. Because alcoholism has been most thoroughly researched, most of the review will concern this disorder. The two most crucial factors in the development of alcoholism are a genetic predisposition and reinforcements coming from the social environment.

Chapter 13 focuses on eating disorders. Although anorexia nervosa and bulimia nervosa each have biological predispositions, these disorders are not seen with any frequency except under specific social conditions.

Chapter 14 examines three important disorders arising in childhood or adolescence. Attention-deficit/hyperactivity disorder is an example of a disorder rooted in a widely distributed trait. Conduct disorder is unique in psychiatry in that it is largely environmental in origin, although predispositions are involved in cases that go on to become adult criminality. Autistic disorder is an example of a disease that was once thought to be environmental in origin but has now been shown to be associated with strong genetic factors.

Chapter 15 examines personality disorders. These conditions have often been considered to be primarily due to environmental stressors. However, research now shows that genetic factors, reflected by variations in personality traits, constitute crucial predispositions. Psychosocial factors remain important as stressors, amplifying underlying traits to the pathological levels that lead to dysfunction.

The last two chapters in this volume address the broader implications of predisposition–stress theory.

Chapter 16 discusses how the predisposition–stress model can be used to guide psychiatric treatment. In it I address the negative consequences associated with biological and environmental reductionism. Two clinical problems are described that demonstrate each of these problems: the treatment of depression, and the use of psychotherapy in the personality disorders.

Chapter 17 discusses the implications of predisposition–stress theory for the prevention of psychiatric illness. I conclude the chapter by examining how the model encourages a greater use of multivariate research on mental disorders.

▎ Acknowledgments

A book such as this one, which summarizes a vast literature, could not have been written without a good deal of help. I would therefore like to acknowledge some of those who have assisted me in this task. I must, of course, make the customary disclaimer that any mistakes in the text are the entire responsibility of the author.

I benefited greatly from the input of two readers who accepted the labor of reviewing the entire manuscript, both in its early stages and in later versions. My wife, Rosalind Paris, helped me to organize the book in a coherent way, and pointed out, with admirable persistence, each case in which I had expressed myself obscurely, suggesting ways to make my ideas clearer. My longtime research colleague Hallie Zweig-Frank was, as always, helpful in pointing out where my thoughts failed to follow logically from each other, and where I had failed to explain fully to the reader ideas that I take for granted. (I would also like to thank Herta Guttman, who read large portions of the text and provided a critical appraisal of my overall conclusions.)

In view of the specialized nature of the literature reviewed here, it was also important to have earlier drafts of these chapters read by experts who were highly knowledgeable about specific areas. For this purpose, I asked for help from several friends and colleagues at McGill University. Peter Hechtman read the chapters on genetics and medical illness and helped me to clarify these complex issues. Heinz Lehmann provided critiques of the chapters on schizophrenia and mood disorders. Maurice Dongier helped me to revise the chapter on substance disorders. Howard Steiger critically reviewed the chapter on eating disorders. Lillie Hechtman provided a detailed critique of the chapter on disorders arising in childhood.

Chapter 15, on the personality disorders, is a heavily revised version of a theory developed in several books and journal articles (Paris 1994, 1996a, 1996b, 1996c).

I would like to acknowledge those who provided the time required to write the text: the Department of Psychiatry of the Sir Mortimer B. Davis–Jewish General Hospital, and its Psychiatrist in Chief, Dr. Phillip Beck; and the Department of Psychiatry of McGill University, and its former Chairman, Dr. Gilbert Pinard. The librarians at the Institute of Community and Family Psychiatry, Ruth Stillman and Judy Grossman, were indispensable in obtaining references. John Oldham, who read the original proposal of this book, provided heartening encouragement for the validity of my ideas.

Few authors get very far without the help of good editors. Carol Nadelson and the editorial staff at American Psychiatric Press have helped me to shape this book, to improve its accuracy, and to focus the text to reach its intended audience.

The dedicatee of this book is, by any standard, a giant in contemporary psychiatry. Sir Michael Rutter is both a great theorist and a great researcher. He has been responsible for a large number of seminal ideas about the causes of mental disorders, and has studied both genetic and environmental factors in development. Inevitably, he is quoted many times in this volume. Although he will, most probably, not agree with all of my conclusions, I am deeply indebted to his theoretical perspective, which addresses the true complexity of psychiatry, yet always remains grounded in empirical data.

I would also like to acknowledge my teachers, my colleagues, and my students at McGill University. I am also grateful to the researchers whose findings form the basis of this book.

Finally, I would like to offer special thanks to my wife, Rosalind Paris. Many years ago, she encouraged me to enter psychiatry. Since then, she has continued to provide consistent and much-needed support for my career.

PART I

Theory

Historical Overview

Psychiatry is a house divided. Forty years ago, in a classic study of psychiatric practice in New Haven, Connecticut, Hollingshead and Redlich (1958) described how psychiatrists fell into two categories: "directive–organic" types, who wore white coats and whose therapies consisted mostly of physical treatment, and "analytic–psychological" types, who wore jackets and whose treatment consisted of talking therapy.

Today's clinicians are much more eclectic than those of 40 years ago. Even so, our discipline continues to suffer from ideological divisions. Although everyone accepts in principle the need to consider both nature and nurture, practice is another matter. Some psychiatrists treat patients almost exclusively with drugs. Others remain primarily interested in psychotherapy. These differences in practice derive from different models of the causes of mental illness.

Many clinicians believe that psychiatry is not different from other branches of medicine. In their view, since most forms of psychopathology derive from biological aberrations, clinicians should use biological methods to correct them. Other clinicians believe that since symptoms emerge from life experiences, therapists should concentrate on helping patients to work through the impact of personal histories. It is ironic that this split continues to bedevil us today, at a time when we know more than ever about the causes of mental disorders and have much more effective ways to treat them. Ultimately, the differences between biological and psychosocial ideas in psychiatry are not really based on evidence. Rather, they are rooted in *ideology*.

Ideas about the etiology of mental disorders often mirror larger intellectual questions. The split within psychiatry reflects another dichotomy that has long been a subject of interest for both philosophers and social scientists: the *nature-versus-nurture dilemma*. This question concerns the extent to which human nature is determined by genes and the extent to which it is shaped by the environment. Over time, theories taking one side or the other of this controversy have influenced the theory and practice of psychiatry. In the present chapter, therefore, we will undertake a historical overview, outlining how these models have influenced clinicians over the last 200 years.

▓ Psychiatry in the 19th Century

In the course of the 19th century, a discipline called "psychiatry" arose out of general medicine (Mora 1975; Shorter 1997). Most of its practitioners were based in mental hospitals, where the majority of the patients suffered from psychotic illnesses. The strongly biological perspective of these early practitioners was therefore quite natural. In fact, psychiatry in the 19th century resembled the ideology of medicine as a whole. Although it was generally acknowledged that the etiology of mental illness was unknown, most clinicians assumed that, as had been the case for other medical diseases, it was only a matter of time before physiological causes would be found.

A number of attempts were made to identify these physiological factors. However, psychiatrists in the previous century were largely unsuccessful in finding biological abnormalities in psychotic patients. (The one dramatic exception was the identification of general paresis as a tertiary manifestation of syphilitic infection.) In retrospect, we can see that this failure was inevitable, given the primitive state of neurobiology at the time. But the inability of a purely medical model to provide a coherent explanation for psychopathology led to widely divergent theories.

In spite of their overall biological bias, clinicians in the 19th century had an intense interest in the psychological factors in mental illness and actively practiced several forms of psychotherapy (Ellenberger 1970). Beginning with the time of Philippe Pinel and the "moral treatment" of the insane, many psychiatrists attempted to apply a psychosocial approach to the treatment of psychotic patients. Hospitals affiliated with universities, such as the Salpêtrière in Paris and the Bürgholzi in Zurich, were particularly active in promoting this psychological approach to mental illness.

The psychiatric paradigms of the late 19th century are well reflected in the work of the German psychiatrist Emil Kraepelin (1919). In his own time, Kraepelin was undoubtedly the world's most respected theorist on mental illness. His ideas have again become strongly influential in contemporary thinking, leading to the formation of a "neo-Kraepelinian" school (Klerman 1986). Although Kraepelin has been criticized for a purported lack of humanism (Laing 1967), he stood for principles that have remained at the core of our discipline: a focus on the phenomenology of mental illness, a hard-headed empiricism, a refusal to make unnecessary speculations, and a resistance to invoking constructs that cannot be operationalized and measured.

Nature and Nurture in 20th-Century Psychiatry

At the end of the 19th century, mainstream psychiatry continued to be based on the observation of psychotic patients. This approach was unsatisfactory to a younger generation, who wanted to work in innovative and creative ways with a broader population. In this context, the new discipline of psychoanalysis attracted many clinicians, both medical and nonmedical.

Most practicing analysts did not work in hospitals, but treated populations of neurotic outpatients in offices and clinics. Psychoanalytic theory offered not only a new way to understand psychopathology but also a general theory of human psychology (Gellner 1993). The new treatment method generated enthusiasm for its therapeutic potential. Psychodynamic ideas also had enormous influence outside formal analysis, both on the general practice of psychotherapy and on the culture as a whole (Hale 1995).

The institutional structure of psychoanalysis encouraged the spread of its influence. Freud's decision to create separate pedagogical institutions to promote his ideas encouraged practitioners to make their primary allegiance psychoanalysis rather than medicine. In fact, many of the early analysts were psychologists or teachers. Moreover, particularly in America, psychoanalysts aimed to influence practice among their nonanalytic colleagues.

Between the First and Second World Wars, biological and psychological models contended for the soul of psychiatry. The biological camp could not yet offer adequate treatments for the major psychoses, even though its defenders devised a number of interesting experimental therapies. (The only Nobel Prizes in medicine ever awarded to doctors working with psychiatric patients were awarded to an Austrian neurologist, Wagner-Jauregg, for the malaria treatment of syphilis, and to a Portuguese neurosurgeon, Moniz, for the development of psychosurgery.)

After World War II, psychiatry was as divided into two camps: those who conformed to a medical model and provided organic treatments, and psychoanalysts, who were committed to the "talking cure." On the biological side of the divide, electroconvulsive therapy (ECT) was being greatly overused. This therapy, which eventually found its place as an effective treatment for melancholia, was, in the absence of effective drugs, being prescribed for all forms of depression. Insulin therapy was also a popular method, although it was later discarded when clinical trials failed to demonstrate its effectiveness (Mora 1975). Psychosurgery was another psychiatric "fad" that later become almost entirely discredited (Valenstein 1986). It was not until the 1950s, with the development of neuroleptics and tricyclic antidepressants, that effective biological treatment became a reality.

On the psychological side of the divide, psychoanalysis reached the zenith of its influence in the 1950s and 1960s. At that time, being an analyst was almost a "must" qualification to become a chairman of academic departments of psychiatry (Eisenberg 1995). Yet even at its time of greatest dominance, psychoanalysis was itself divided. The movement has always had a tendency to splinter, and many variants of Freud's original model existed. Among the forms of psychotherapy common in the 1960s were "neo-Freudian" forms of analysis, client-centered therapy, group therapy, and family therapy. Still, most of these offshoots remained far closer intellectually to psychoanalysis than to organic psychiatry. As different as these ideas were, all of them had one important thing in common: they were rooted in theories attributing psychopathology primarily to psychosocial factors (Paris 1973).

Today, this picture has greatly changed. As in the 19th century, many psychiatrists have adopted biological theories of mental illness. The fact that we now have pharmacological agents that are highly effective and that have relatively few side effects has had a profound effect on the way clinicians think. With so many disorders correctable with medication, clinicians are much more tempted to espouse theories reducing psychopathology to "chemical imbalances."

Psychotherapies today have a much narrower scope than they once did. One reason for the decline of psychotherapy is that it was oversold, leading to disappointment and disillusionment (Eisenberg 1995). Although psychotherapeutic methods have been shown by empirical research to be effective for a wide variety of patients (Bergin and Garfield 1994), they often work more slowly than drugs, and they are relatively ineffective for patients with severe psychopathology.

Reductionism in Contemporary Psychiatry

Psychiatric models have had an unfortunate history of moving from one extreme to another. Grinker (1964) described the unbridled enthusiasm for community psychiatry that characterized the 1960s in a memorable phrase, "psychiatry rushes off in all directions." Today, more than 30 years later, we are still searching for the right direction.

Biological psychiatrists have been insufficiently interested in studying the psychological precipitants of mental disorders. In a witty comment, Lipowski (1989) suggested that whereas the era in which psychodynamic psychiatry predominated was characterized by "brainlessness," the contemporary biological era is characterized by "mindlessness." There is a real danger that contemporary psychiatrists will lose interest in "the person." This would be a tragic outcome of the great achievements of modern biological research. No matter how sophisticated we become in studying the brain, when we stop talking to our patients, we lose the soul of our profession. Moreover, we cannot fully understand the origins of mental disorders through biological correlates. As wise physicians have always known, all illnesses have a unique course, shaped by the events of patients' lives.

At the same time, few psychotherapists have taken the implications of genetic research into account in their work. Most clinicians accept that certain illnesses, particularly schizophrenia and bipolar disorder, have a strong genetic component. Unfortunately, this information is often kept in a "compartment," allowing clinicians to believe that *other* forms of mental disorder are largely psychological.

As will be shown in this book, biological factors are involved in the development of almost *all* forms of pathology, even including conditions, such as posttraumatic stress disorder and personality disorders, that have often been considered to be primarily environmental in origin.

Unfortunately, much of the psychotherapeutic community continues to subscribe to an environmentally reductionistic paradigm, explaining psychic distress as a reaction to events during childhood. These clinicians are ignoring the genetic and biological factors underlying even the most common psychological symptoms.

The ebb and flow of scientific ideas is not, of course, determined only by fashion. In the long run, theories must stand or fall on the weight of cumulative empirical evidence (Kuhn 1970). Nevertheless, in the short run, there is some relationship between theoretical preferences and cultural values.

Environmentalist ideas have had their most powerful impact in North America. This may not be a coincidence. J. Frank and J. B. Frank (1991) have suggested sociological reasons for the differences between American and European ideas. They point out that American society deeply values individualism and promotes the belief that individual goals should not be shackled—not by tradition and not by biological imperatives. On the other hand, Europe retains a relatively more traditional way of life. Thus, even today, European psychiatry continues to be strongly influenced by theories that emphasize the constitutional factors in mental illness.

On this side of the Atlantic, a disparate range of environmentalist theories have been influential, including certain schools of psychoanalysis, classical behaviorism, and social models of mental illness. In recent years, theories accounting for adult symptoms on the basis of childhood trauma have had a strong impact on clinicians as well as the general public. What all these environmental models have in common is that they attribute the etiology of mental disorders almost entirely to psychological and social factors: traumatic life events, bad families, or a "sick society."

There is nonetheless a grain of truth in these ideas. As will be discussed later in this book, there is empirical evidence that traumatic life events increase the risk for many forms of psychopathology. There is evidence that dysfunctional families are more likely to produce children with mental disorders. And there is evidence that levels of social cohesion affect the prevalence of psychiatric illness.

However, what environmental models fail to take into account is that these associations between risk factors and psychopathology are only statistical. In other words, more people who are exposed to risks will fall ill, but most do not. The effects of the environment depend on factors within the person. Even the most pathogenic environmental stressors do not produce disorders in the absence of predispositions.

Scarr (1991), in a discussion of why the genetic factors in intelligence and personality are dismissed by many people, asked:

> Why the resistance to the idea that parents transmit genes to their children, with the consequence that their children resemble them to a modest extent? Because behavioral scientists understand genetic transmission to mean that nothing can be done to change the unfortunate lot of people who inherit bad genes. (p. 385)

As social opportunities become more equal, individual differences tend to stand out even more dramatically. As Scarr (1991) has emphasized, "egalitarian provisions *raise* the heritability of personal and intellectual characteristics in Western populations" (p. 386 [emphasis added]).

An understanding of predispositions can help us to take a more humane view of mental illness. When we recognize that patients have inherent areas of vulnerability, we will hold neither them nor those in their immediate environment entirely responsible for their problems. When we treat patients, we need to provide them with whatever forms of treatment have been shown to be effective, without being in any way judgmental. For this reason, acknowledging the genetic factors in mental disorders need not lead to determinism or despair, but can instead be the basis of a higher form of humanism.

2

Genetic Predispositions to Disease

All organisms are biologically programmed to survive and reproduce. A master plan coded in the genes shapes all phenotypic traits, including anatomical structures, physiological functioning, and behaviors. These programs are laid down in two types of genes: a smaller number that code for the synthesis of specific proteins, and a larger number that regulate the development of fertilized eggs into complex organisms.

Although most human characteristics have a genetic component, there is no simple correspondence between genes and traits. As pointed out by Pinker (1994),

a single gene rarely specifies some identifiable part of an organism. Instead it specifies the release of a protein at specific times in development, an ingredient of an unfathomably complex recipe, usually in having some effect in molding a suite of parts that are affected by other genes. (pp. 321–322)

Thus, even when, over the next few decades, we succeed in decoding the human genome, we will still be a long way from being able to describe how changes at the level of the genetic code shape phenotypes. Understanding the genetic factors behind behavioral traits will present particularly thorny difficulties. As Pinker (1994) puts it,

> the relationship between particular genes and particular psychological traits is doubly indirect. First, a single gene does not build a single brain module; the brain is a delicately layered soufflé in which each gene product is an ingredient with a complex effect on many properties of many circuits. Second, a single brain module does not produce a single behavioral trait. Most of the traits which capture our attention emerge out of unique combinations of kinks in many different modules. (p. 328)

Human behavior is not, therefore, controlled by heredity like a puppet on a genetic string. Genes code for proteins, not behaviors. Thus, there is no such thing as a gene "for shyness," a gene "for criminality," or a gene "for homosexuality." Rather, each of these psychological traits is influenced by interactions between many gene loci and between genes and the environment.

The relationship between complex traits and phenotypes is enormously complex. We often observe "genetic heterogeneity," in which the same outcome can emerge from different combinations of genes. In addition, the same combinations of genes can lead to different outcomes. It needs to emphasized that the expression of genes can be different under different environmental conditions. Many genes are inoperative unless they are "turned on" by the environment. Thus, even if we had a complete map of the human genome, we would not be able to make precise predictions of phenotypes in any individual (Lewontin 1992).

In summary, the following principles describe the relationship of genes to behavior:

1. Predispositions for behavior are usually not expressed without the presence of a complex combination of genetic factors.
2. Some sets of behaviors reflect strong genetic factors, whereas other behaviors are under weak genetic influence.

3. Even when significant genetic predispositions for behavioral traits are present, environmental factors are usually required to make them manifest.

Evolution and Human Disease

Natural selection is a mechanism that maximizes fitness to the environment. What evolutionary theory means by "fitness" is the extent to which genes affect the likelihood that organisms successfully reproduce. This leads to a paradoxical question: given that genes are a product of natural selection, why do pathogenic genetic variants remain in the population?

Nesse and Williams (1994) have provided the best account of why, if genes are programmed to maximize fitness, we remain prone to disease. Two basic explanations account for genetic vulnerability to illness. First, natural selection acts only on those characteristics that influence reproductive capacity. Genes that increase the likelihood of developing diseases prior to or during the reproductive years will tend to be selected out of the population. At the same time, genes that lead to disease only later in life can remain in the gene pool, since genes that express themselves only *after* reproduction are immune to natural selection.

A well-known example of this principle is Huntington's disease. This illness is caused by a dominant gene associated with the presence of an abnormal genetic sequence termed "trinucleotide repeats." Once the disease begins, usually in middle age, it is incurable and eventually fatal. Yet, since the gene has no effect in the reproductive years, Huntington's disease is transmitted to offspring and remains in the population.

The second reason we remain vulnerable to disease is that body plans developed by evolution are not perfect. Every species has inborn protective mechanisms against disease. However, there is a balance in natural selection between the effectiveness of a protection and its cost to the organism. Most aspects of organismic design represent compromises between these conflicting forces. For example, the large and complex human brain brings many selective advantages, but is also associated with significant costs, such as high levels of morbidity during childbirth. Moreover, some genetic effects are accidents of history, "pleiomorphic" traits that were selected for another purpose but that lead to incidental and unanticipated consequences (Gould and Lewontin 1979).

The process of *aging* itself might be due to both of these processes: accumulated genetic effects acting later in the life cycle, and intrinsic design flaws in the organism. These factors may explain why senescence is biologically inevitable (Nesse and Williams 1994). Yet, genetically determined diseases frequently affect young people. To understand why, we need to review the mechanisms of genetic transmission.

The gene pool in any population is subject to a constant process of mutation. Most of these mutations reduce fitness and are therefore quickly selected out of the population. Those rare mutations that increase fitness can fire the engine of evolution.

Genetic variations in any trait can be positive, negative, or neutral, depending on environmental conditions. For example, genes increasing rates of fat storage are adaptive under conditions of famine but maladaptive when food is abundant (see Chapter 13). Thus, characteristics that evolved for adaptation in one environment can be maladaptive in a different environment.

In classic Mendelian heredity, traits are essentially either "on" or "off." However, in some cases of recessive inheritance, heterozygotes can still be affected by an abnormal trait, albeit less severely than homozygotes. In certain diseases, there may even be a selective advantage to heterozygosity, with the result that the genes involved are more likely to remain in the population. This phenomenon is termed "balanced polymorphism."

The mechanism of this effect is best exemplified by sickle cell anemia. Although this disease is severe and life-threatening, the gene for the trait remains common in black populations. The reason is that heterozygosity for the condition—in which the red blood cells assume a crescent shape that makes it more difficult for the parasite (*Plasmodium malariae*) to survive—protects carriers against malaria, which is highly endemic in Africa. However, in the malaria-free North American environment, heterozygosity, leading to moderate sickling of red cells, conveys no advantage, while the massive sickling seen in homozygous individuals leads to serious illness.

Although this example is taught to every biology student, few other clear-cut cases of balanced polymorphism have been found. Speculations that heterozygosity for genetic diseases such as cystic fibrosis or Gaucher's disease might protect against other types of illness (Nesse and Williams 1994) have not been supported by convincing evidence.

In summary, diseases remain in the population for several reasons. Diseases with dominant Mendelian inheritance may begin late in life or may reemerge as the result of spontaneous mutations. Diseases with recessive Mendelian inheritance remain in the population because carriers are less severely affected. Diseases with a polygenic, non-Mendelian inheritance involve many gene loci, each of which is insufficient to cause illness, thus effectively reducing the pressure of natural selection.

Genetic Mechanisms and Human Disease

We all fall ill, but with different diseases. Our genes play a crucial role in determining which illnesses we are most likely to contract.

Genetic epidemiology (Falconer 1989) is a discipline that uses studies of large populations to examine the interactions of genes and environment in the etiology of disease. Genetics has traditionally been concerned only with biological factors, while epidemiology has focused on the environmental factors in disease. Genetic epidemiology, in contrast, has the goal of combining both in a single discipline, elucidating the mechanisms by which environmental factors determine the pathways from predispositions to pathology.

Faraone and Tsuang (1995) have described several stages in the study of the genetic factors in medical illness: 1) examining whether a disease runs in families; 2) determining the relative contributions of genes and environment to its etiology; 3) establishing whether there is a specific pattern of inheritance; 4) attempting to locate on specific chromosomes those genes that can influence the development of disease; and 5) determining the physiological and biochemical mechanisms by which genes act to cause disease.

This chapter will review some of the research methods used to elucidate these genetic mechanisms. Since the focus of this book is on understanding gene–environment interactions, we will first address the question of *why* traits show strong individual differences. We will then examine *patterns of inheritance* affecting these differences. Finally, we will review the methods that can *quantitatively* estimate the heritability of any trait or illness.

■ Explaining Individual Differences

Human beings differ greatly one from another. They look different, have different intellectual capacities, demonstrate different personality traits, and suffer from different diseases. Moreover, individual differences in personality traits are associated with differential vulnerabilities to mental disorders (Krueger et al. 1996). A comprehensive theory of psychopathology must therefore take these variations into account.

Individual differences can result from nature or nurture. Biologists tend to focus on nature, whereas social scientists prefer to emphasize nurture. However, the interactions of nature and nurture provide the most adequate explanation of why individuals differ from each other.

With the exception of monozygotic twins, none of us have exactly the same genes. Even if we could fully map the human genome, the precise location of each set of base pairs would be slightly different in everyone. This is why we all begin life with different traits. Genetic differences also impose limits on the forms environmentally induced expressions can take. However, individual differences in traits can be either *amplified* or *suppressed* by the environment.

A good example of *amplification* is the relationship between personality traits and personality disorders (see Chapter 15). Each type of personality is potentially adaptive, and individual differences need not be in any way pathogenic (Beck and Freeman 1990). Yet these traits, when amplified to dysfunctional levels, can cause significant psychopathology. Dysfunction becomes most likely when traits are exaggerated and when they are not buffered by interactions with more adaptive traits.

The basic dimensions of personality, such as extraversion and introversion, are normal variants in any population. However, even these traits can become problematic, either because they are unusually intense or because environmental factors lead to their amplification. Thus, within a normal range, extraverts are charming and attractive people. However, at a certain point, it becomes dysfunctional to be excessively extraverted, particularly if it makes one excessively dependent on the responses of others. Similarly, introversion is normally functional and is associated with a useful self-sufficiency. However, amplification of this trait can lead to social isolation.

Intelligence provides an interesting example of the *suppression* of genetic differences. As will be discussed in Chapter 5, there are large differences in concordance between monozygotic and dizygotic twins on IQ tests, evidence providing strong support for the heritability of intellectual capacities. Yet these differences are not seen when socially disadvantaged twins, such as black Americans, are compared with each other (Scarr 1981). The most likely reason is that strong environmental factors lower IQ scores in many members of this population, "flattening out" underlying genetic differences.

Patterns of Inheritance

The inheritance of most human diseases is non-Mendelian and polygenic. Each predisposition to illness is based not on single genes but on interactions between many genes (Falconer 1989). Some of these genes have major effects, while others may have only minor effects. Because predispositions to illness depend on cumulative polygenic effects, many of these genes remain in the population, since, by themselves, they may have no pathogenic consequences.

The development of most diseases also depends on interactions between the genes and the environment. This phenomenon has been called "penetrance" or "variable expressivity." Environmental factors can be the main determinants of whether a predisposition remains latent or leads to overt illness. For each predisposed individual who falls ill, there will be many others who develop no illness at all or who develop only a subclinical form of illness.

We will provide many examples of the principles of gene–environment interactions in the coming chapters, both in medical and psychiatric illness. At this point, we might briefly consider the example of adult-onset diabetes mellitus. The genes that constitute the predisposition to diabetes are widely distributed in the population but cause disease only when there is an adequate food supply (MacDonald 1988). In the environments in which humanity evolved, the diabetic gene might actually have protected its carriers from starvation by allowing for a more rapid breakdown of fat stores. In our present environment of abundance, the same genes may cause disease. Thus, in Native American cultures, the prevalence of diabetes, related to abundant food supplies, has dramatically risen (MacDonald 1988). This relationship also explains why many diabetic patients can be treated simply by restricting the number of calories in their diets.

Measuring Heritability

Heritability is a quantitative estimate of the extent to which any trait is inherited. The measurement of heritability has a long and distinguished history in medical research. Studies can be conducted in either community or clinical samples, but findings drawn from population-based research are more broadly generalizable than those drawn from clinical samples, which are usually biased in one way or another.

Family History Studies

Family history is the classical method of studying heritability. The first step involves constructing pedigrees to determine whether a trait or disorder runs in families. The second step involves "segregation analysis," i.e., determining whether the pattern of transmission within the pedigree conforms to a Mendelian model (Elston and Stewart 1971). There are two limitations to the family history method. The first is that there is no clear way to separate genetic from environmental factors. The second is that pedigree studies are drawn only from families with affected members, rather than from the general population, and the findings are therefore strictly applicable only to this group.

Nonetheless, whenever family history studies have suggested that disorders are genetic, twin or adoption studies have confirmed the assumption of heritability (Andreasen et al. 1986). The presence of a positive family history of any disorder can therefore be regarded as strongly presumptive of genetic factors.

Pedigree studies are important for another reason. Although genetic predispositions may or may not express themselves as overt disease, we can find markers for their presence in the unaffected relatives of individuals who develop overt illness. Each genetic variation is associated with some change in physiology and/or biochemistry. When many genes are involved in the inheritance of an illness, each one of them can be associated with a measurable biological change. We can use the pedigrees of patients with specific disorders to search for these markers.

Twin Studies

The heritability of any trait can be calculated from differences in concordances for a trait between monozygotic (MZ) and dizygotic (DZ) twins. A finer-grained procedure for determining whether traits are heritable is called "model fitting." This procedure is used to test how well several different models (genetic, environmental, or mixed genetic–environmental) account for the differences between MZ and DZ twins. The variance accounted for by genetic factors can also be apportioned, expressed as a percentage. Finally, computer modeling allows the separation of two types of genetic effects, "additive" and "nonadditive." Effects are said to be additive if a number of genetic factors add more or less equal increments to the phenotype. Nonadditive effects, in contrast, reflect the presence of a major Mendelian gene that is responsible for a large percentage of the trait variance, although the influence of this single locus is ordinarily modified by interactions with other genes.

There are two caveats to keep in mind about the interpretation of twin studies. First, it is misleading to think that "heritability," expressed as a percentage, reflects the precise strength of genetic influence in any one person. Rather, it measures the extent to which individual differences in a trait within a population can be accounted for by genes. Thus, heritability estimates do not apply to individuals, in whom genes or environment can have greater or lesser contributions to outcome, but to group means. In other words, different individuals can have greater or lesser genetic contributions to the same trait. Second, the percentage of variance attributable to heredity depends on the population under study. Since the ultimate effects of genes depend on their interactions with the environment, the same trait can have different degrees of heritability in different socioeconomic groups or in different societies.

Other questions that have been raised about the validity of twin studies are of less concern. Much of the criticism of twin-study methodology has been rather tendentious—there are at least as many problems in interpreting studies of the nongenetic factors in disease. First, there are no unique characteristics in twins that are not found in nontwins (Kendler et al. 1993d). Second, a wide body of data (Kendler et al. 1993d; Plomin 1994a) supports the "equal environments assumption" that there are only minor differences in the rearing of identical and fraternal twins by parents. This assumption has been shown to hold for a number of psychiatric disorders (Kendler et al. 1993d). Actually, twins raised apart are *more* similar than those raised together (Shields 1962), probably because twins who are raised together try to maximize their differences (Plomin 1994a).

One of the most interesting applications of twin methodology is in estimating the *environmental* factors affecting human traits (Kendler 1995; Plomin 1994b). In addition to determining the percentage of genetic influence on individual differences for any trait, we can calculate the influence of two types of environmental factors. The first type—the *shared environment*—depends on similarities between individuals associated with living in the same family. The second type is the *unshared environment*. This residual variance has many sources. It probably reflects differences in experiences within the same family, or differential niches for siblings (Sulloway 1996), as well as the effects of life experiences outside the family (Reiss et al. 1992).

Behavioral genetics is a discipline applying twin-study methods to the study of genetic and environmental factors in behavioral traits such as intelligence and personality. As we will see in Chapter 5, intelligence has a large genetic component. Behavioral genetic studies of personality are of particular interest, since personality traits are crucial factors in understanding the origins of mental disorders.

Millon and Davis (1995) have compared personality to an immune system that processes environmental stimuli of all kinds. In addition to constituting predispositions to personality disorders (see Chapter 15), personality traits are important predisposing factors for major psychiatric illnesses (Cloninger 1987; Krueger et al. 1996). Genetic factors account for nearly half of the variance in personality traits (Plomin 1994a). This is the case for the broader dimensions of personality as well as for most narrowly defined traits.

Even the environmental factors influencing behavior are partly a function of the genes. Thus, genetically controlled traits shape a child's intellectual environment, so that intelligent children gravitate toward experiences that facilitate intellectual development (Scarr and McCartney 1983). Moreover, since the manner in which we respond to environmental challenges depends on our personality traits, genes influence the overall quality of our life experiences (see Chapter 3).

Adoption Studies

Studies of adopted children are particularly useful in overcoming the problem of confounding genetic and environmental factors in disease. If adoptees are more similar to their biological parents than to their adoptive parents, this provides very strong evidence indeed for heritability of a trait. Studies of both intelligence and personality traits (Plomin 1994a) demonstrate that adopted children and their biological parents have similarities in many traits. Studies of psychiatric disorders in adopted subjects have almost always yielded findings that parallel those of twin studies.

Most criticisms of adoption study methodology (e.g., Lidz and Blatt 1983) can be easily dismissed (Plomin 1994a). Thus, there is no evidence that the process by which children are placed has an effect on behavior, or that the psychological effects of adoption itself lead to major pathogenic effects. These objections can hardly explain data showing that biological children of a schizophrenic mother are more likely to develop schizophrenia, even when raised by adoptive parents without mental illness.

The study of twins separated at birth combines the advantages of twin study and adoption study methods. Although such studies provide a powerful way to measure heritability, cases are understandably few. However, a large-scale project conducted at the University of Minnesota collected subjects from all over the United States. The results of this study were widely reported in the media, often punctuated by picturesque anecdotes exemplifying surprising similarities between separated twins. The quantitative findings of this study strongly supported earlier research that showed dramatic similarities in both intelligence and personality between twins reared apart (Bouchard et al. 1990; Lykken et al. 1992; Tellegen et al. 1988).

Biological Markers

The search for biological markers for disease is one of the major thrusts of contemporary medical research. When a marker is consistently associated with a disorder, it strongly suggests the existence of underlying genetic factors. However, since biological markers may reflect only the secondary effects of disease, they need not always have etiological significance. To make this distinction, we need to know whether the marker was present before the disorder developed, or whether it is a result of a pathological process initiated by the disorder.

Psychiatrists would eventually like to be able to make diagnoses much in the same way as internists, confirming their clinical impressions by conducting laboratory tests. Thus far, the search for markers *specific* to mental disorders has been rather frustrating. Some of the most promising measures, such as platelet monoamine oxidase activity (Buchsbaum and Haier 1983) and dexamethasone suppression (F. K. Goodwin and Jamieson 1990), have turned out to have a nonspecific relationship to psychopathology. In spite of enormous research efforts in schizophrenia, no markers specific to that disorder have been found (Gottesman 1991).

There are two possible explanations for the lack of a definite relationship between neurochemical or neurophysiological findings and specific mental disorders. First and foremost, even in this "decade of the brain," we know little about how that organ actually works. Current technology is highly complex and impressive, particularly imaging techniques that allow us to study the brain in vivo. Yet succeeding generations may view these efforts as primitive. Thus, even though our theories about the biological bases of behavior are becoming much more sophisticated, future psychiatrists may see our models as simplistic. Second, biological markers are usually more strongly related to the traits that underlie disease than to overt disorders (Siever and Davis 1991). In other words, *diseases do not constitute phenotypes.* Every disease may represent a rare form of a widely distributed trait. Outcomes are dependent on environmental factors, and genetic vulnerability may or may not lead to disease. This could be the main reason that illness-specific biological markers have not often been found.

Genetic Mapping

Ultimately, the role of genes in human illness will be elucidated through the complete mapping of the human genome (Billings et al. 1992; Weissenbach et al. 1992). Ideally, we will then be able to associate predispositions to disease with specific genetic variations at one or (more likely) several sites. In this scenario, we would be in a position to identify individual predispositions to disease before illnesses actually develop.

Achieving this goal will not, however, be easy. There are about 30 billion base pairs in the human genome. The number of genes is considerably lower than that, probably about 100,000. Linking any one gene, or several genes, to a disease will involve searching for needles in many haystacks.

However, while we await the mapping of the genome, we can use two other methods. *Genetic association* involves gathering data showing that changes at gene loci are associated with specific diseases. *Genetic linkage* involves finding precise chromosomal locations of genes associated with disease or with predispositions to disease. Linkage analysis (Faraone and Tsuang 1995) often depends on the possibility that a trait under study is on the same chromosome and lies close to the locus of a known genetic marker, such as human leukocyte antigens (HLAs). Even in the absence of such known markers, linkage studies can take advantage of the fact that pieces of chromosomes "cross over" during meiosis, so that when two genes are particularly close to each other, they remain linked, even when they end up on different chromosomes. Technological improvements are rapidly increasing the number of identified gene loci for disease.

One outgrowth of linkage analysis is the sibling-pair method (for an example, see McBride and Anderson 1996). This approach is particularly useful when the mode of inheritance is unknown and when many gene loci are involved. Siblings would ordinarily be expected to share genes about half the time, but if two siblings are both affected by the same illness and if the sharing of a marker is above the chance rate, then this region of the chromosome may contain a gene associated with susceptibility to the disease under study.

The availability of large family pedigrees of affected individuals makes these type of studies much more practical. It is often of particular importance to determine whether the same genes are present in unaffected relatives; such a finding would indicate that the predisposition to a disease is more widely distributed than the overt illness. In the last 15 years, many of the advances in medical genetics have depended on these linkage studies.

Massive research efforts are now under way to determine genetic linkages for many major medical disorders. Thus far, some of the best-known diseases that have been linked to specific gene loci include cystic fibrosis, Huntington's disease, Friedreich's ataxia, neurofibromatosis, and myotonic dystrophy (Faraone and Tsuang 1995).

There have been, thus far, no firm findings linking the major mental disorders to gene loci. The one major exception is Alzheimer's disease, in which a marker for genetic vulnerability has been found in early-onset cases (Corder et al. 1993). As a result of the excitement about gene mapping, we often read in newspapers about the latest research supporting one "candidate gene" or another. Unfortunately, in most cases, findings in one sample fail to be confirmed in other samples. This should not be a cause for discouragement. Even though we do not yet have firm gene loci for mental disorders, we are bound to find them eventually, probably within the next decade. When this happens, both research and practice in psychiatry will undergo dramatic changes (Plomin and Rutter, in press).

■ The Threshold Model of Disease

Most of us usually consider people as either sick or well; we are accustomed to thinking of health and illness as a dichotomy. Yet in most cases there is a *continuum* between health and illness. We all carry around within ourselves a set of liabilities—genetic potentials to develop specific diseases—that become activated in the presence of stressful environmental factors.

When diseases are caused by single genes with a Mendelian pattern of inheritance, the relationship between traits and disorder will be more or less *dichotomous*—that is, either individuals will have a disease or they will not. In contrast, predispositions caused by multiple genes are quantitative, and therefore much more likely to cause a *continuous* distribution of variations, with no sharp break between traits and disorders.

In most chronic diseases, predispositions depend on multiple genes as well as on multiple environmental risks. This complexity creates a continuity between health and illness. Depending on how many pathogenic genes are activated, the weight of biological predispositions will vary from one person to another. Therefore, some individuals, with a stronger genetic weighting, are likely to develop illness with little or no environmental provocation. Others, with a weaker predisposition, may only develop illness if exposed to relatively severe environmental stressors.

Traits and disorders cannot, therefore, be clearly separated. Disorders become diagnosable at a cutoff point at which underlying traits interfere with functioning. A familiar clinical example of this principle is hypertension. Multiple genes are involved in the predisposition to this disease (Falconer 1989). Moreover, many environmental factors, ranging from diet to kidney disease, can raise blood pressure. These environmental effects will be much more pathogenic in those who are genetically predisposed to hypertension.

Some thresholds for disease are relatively arbitrary. For example, the traditional cutoff for hypertension (blood pressure greater than 140/90 mm Hg) simply reflects our clinical experience that the secondary complications of hypertension become much more likely somewhere around this point. As we will see in later chapters, a number of psychiatric conditions, from attention-deficit/hyperactivity disorder to personality disorders, are traits that have crossed a threshold at which they are more likely to produce significant dysfunction.

The threshold model of disease can be modeled mathematically (Falconer 1989). The sum of all of the qualitative factors, genetic and environmental, that contribute to the expression of a trait constitute a continuously distributed quantitative measure termed *liability*.

Certain observable characteristics of disease help to determine the nature of this liability. The first concerns the natural history of an illness. Some genetic predispositions have "sleeper" effects that become manifest only later in life (the genetic predisposition to Alzheimer's disease would be an example).

There is an interesting relationship between timing of onset and the strength of genetic weighting in illnesses with a polygenic pattern of inheritance (Childs and Scriver 1986). Early-onset cases tend to have a larger genetic component, while late-onset ones tend to have a larger environmental component. Early-onset cases tend to involve more affected relatives and to be more severe that late-onset cases.

Childs and Scriver (1986) offer illustrations of the principle that timing of onset is a marker for the strength of a genetic predisposition. A variety of chronic diseases are characterized by polygenic inheritance: duodenal ulcer, non–insulin dependent diabetes mellitus, Crohn's disease, and gout. In each of these, an early onset is associated with a stronger family history and more severe illness. As we will see in later chapters, these principles are applicable to many psychiatric disorders.

A second illness feature that could be used as a marker for the nature of predispositions is sex distribution. Childs and Scriver (1986) suggest that when an illness has a skewed sex distribution, the less frequently affected sex will have a stronger family history and more severe illness. This is because when genetic factors are relatively sex-limited, they develop in interaction with hormones. In the absence of hormonal factors, the genes must have greater "penetrance." For example, although systemic lupus erythematosus is more common in females, it is more severe and is associated with a stronger family history in males. In the same way, gout is more common in males but is more severe and involves a stronger family history in females. Mental disorders with a skewed sex distribution, such as depression and substance abuse in adults, as well as several common psychiatric disorders of childhood, show a parallel relationship between gender and strength of liability.

Multiple thresholds for the same disease are possible when the illness has more severe and less severe subtypes (McGuffin and Gottesman 1985). Multiple thresholds can also be interpreted as indicating that there can be two pathways to the same illness, each involving a different degree of genetic loading. The best example of a psychiatric disorder with multiple pathways is depression—the melancholic and psychotic subtypes are associated with different patterns of predispositions and stressors than the less severe forms.

The threshold for any disease is not fixed, but rather is sensitive to the environment. Even in single-gene diseases such as phenylketonuria, the predisposition will cause severe disease with one type of diet but no disease at all with another type of diet. This principle applies with even greater force to multiple-gene diseases.

Just as the genetic factors in disease are multiple, the environmental factors in illness are also multiple and cumulative. Moreover, their effects can only be understood in terms of interactions with genetic predispositions. The same environmental stressors that lead to chronic illness in one person will lead to acute illness in a second person, and to no illness in a third person.

Summary

We can extract the following principles from the literature reviewed in this chapter:

1. Individuals carry the potential to develop one or more forms of illness.
2. Disorders appear when an individual's total liability crosses a given threshold.
3. Genetic loading determines the level of this threshold.
4. Environmental factors often determine whether these thresholds are crossed.

Clearly, genetic factors play a crucial role in the etiology of human disease. This principle has been supported by studies using many different methodologies. However, although the evidence for heritable factors in pathology is strong, it is largely *indirect,* and final proof will depend on finding specific gene polymorphisms and demonstrating the mechanisms by which these variations affect the organism (Faraone and Tsuang 1995). In the coming decades, elucidating the precise biological mechanisms underlying genetic predispositions will be a major focus of medical research.

3

The Role of Environmental Stressors

The environment is of supreme importance in the etiology of mental disorders. However, stressors can only be understood in the context of their interactions with predispositions. To review, the essentials of the predisposition–stress model are as follows:

1. Predisposing genetic factors are necessary but not sufficient conditions for the development of mental disorders.
2. Environmental factors determine whether or not predispositions cross a threshold of liability and develop into disorders.
3. By themselves, stressors are rarely sufficient conditions for the development of mental disorders.
4. Predispositions determine the specific forms taken by psychopathology.

This chapter will present evidence supporting the following principles:

1. Negative experiences in life need not lead to mental disorders. In both childhood and adulthood, resilience is the rule.
2. The primacy of early childhood experience is not supported by empirical research.
3. The effects of stressors are cumulative, with multiple negative events having more long-term effects than single events.
4. The impact of life experiences is mediated by individual vulnerabilities, as expressed through personality traits.
5. Some individuals require high levels of environmental stressors to become ill, whereas others fall ill in response to minimal levels of stress.
6. Social factors are as important as psychological factors in the etiology of mental disorders.

■ Environmental Stressors and Resilience

The prevalence of predispositions to psychopathology is much higher than the prevalence of any specific disorder. As we will see in future chapters, this principle has been demonstrated in schizophrenia, unipolar depression, substance abuse, eating disorders, attention-deficit/hyperactivity disorder, and personality disorders.

In fact, the genetic linkage research strategy described in Chapter 2 is possible only because we can assess predispositions in nonaffected relatives of mentally ill probands. Fortunately, most people go through life carrying predispositions to psychopathology that are never expressed. Usually, only severe and repeated stressors uncover these vulnerabilities.

By definition, stressful events are those that are most likely to produce negative consequences. Stressors, such as conflicts with parents during childhood or troubling life events, can be idiosyncratic to the individual. Alternatively, they can consist of common factors, such as social or economic problems, that affect everyone to different degrees.

Stressful events during childhood have a well-established relationship with later psychopathology (see reviews in Masten and Coatsworth 1995 and Cohler et al. 1995). On the other hand, as will be discussed in detail later, negative events need not produce long-term sequelae. It is particularly important to note that *single* events, although they often cause short-term symptoms, rarely lead to lasting psychopathology. Instead, long-term sequelae become more likely as the number of negative events increases and accumulates (Rutter 1987a).

However strong the relationship between psychological risk factors and pathological outcome, it is only statistical. Many people are affected, but most are not. The ability to emerge relatively unscathed from negative life events is termed *resilience*. One of the most important findings of research in developmental psychopathology is that *resilience is the rule, not the exception*.

This principle helps to explain why only the most consistent adversities break down children's coping mechanisms. Single events, although stressful for children in the short run, need not lead to long-term consequences. Multiple adversities, in contrast, can overcome natural resilience.

Let us consider, as an example, one of the largest-scale studies of children at risk conducted to date, a 30-year follow-up by Werner and Smith (1992). This study examined children born to Hawaiian plantation workers. Although some might assume that poverty is a major risk factor for developing mental disorders, that supposition was not confirmed by this study's findings. In fact, most of the children at risk eventually became fully competent adults.

Werner and Smith (1992) found that the effects of a stressful environment consistently led to adverse sequelae only in a high-risk subgroup (10% of the total cohort). This high-risk group had experienced multiple adversities, such as dysfunction or breakup of the nuclear family or parental mental illness. Moreover, in this subpopulation, the effect of environmental stressors was cumulative, showing a strong relationship between the total number of risk factors and the likelihood of a pathological outcome. About two-thirds of children with multiple adversities eventually developed serious difficulties, most particularly learning problems, delinquency, or major mental disorders. Nevertheless, even in the high-risk group, as many as one-third became successful and competent adults.

These findings are far from unique to the cohort studied by Werner and Smith. Rutter (1987a) reported a very similar relationship between risk factors and outcome in a series of studies of high-risk children in Britain. The finding that resilience is the rule in childhood adversities has been confirmed in a large number of research studies all over the world (Garmezy and Masten 1994). Moreover, as will be discussed in Chapter 11, children are also surprisingly resilient to even the most traumatic events, including sexual or physical abuse.

Resilience also emerges as a crucial factor determining the long-term effects of environmental stressors during adult life (see review in Staudinger et al. 1995). Again, although negative life events increase the likelihood of pathological outcomes and lower thresholds of liability, they do not consistently lead to adverse sequelae. As will be discussed in future chapters, the onset of mental disorders is often associated with recent negative events. Yet no life event by itself predicts the development of psychopathology.

As will be discussed in some detail in Chapter 11, even the most severe stressors of adult life, such as war and natural disasters (e.g., earthquakes, floods), produce psychopathology only in a minority of individuals. These findings constitute striking confirmation that resilience is the rule in human life. As with children, the effects of stress in adulthood are cumulative, in that the more negative events occur, the more likely the person is to fall ill.

Finally, we need to take into account individual variations in how events are experienced as stressful. The effects of stressors are always processed through personality, so that different people attach different valences of negativity to different events (Rutter and Maughan 1997). Research on the effects of life events, such as major transitions and changes, has consistently demonstrated these differences in relation both to medical illnesses and to psychiatric disorders (Rahe 1995).

The fact that the degree to which any environmental event is stressful varies a great deal among individuals helps to explain why there are very few *specific* relationships between environmental stressors and psychiatric illness. In fact, the relationship between stress and most mental disorders is usually *nonspecific*. The same illness can be brought on by a variety of stressors, and the same stressors can bring on a wide variety of illnesses.

What are the mechanisms behind resilience? Some of these factors are constitutional. The construct of "constitution" consists of two elements: the presence (or absence) of traits that reflect genetic vulnerabilities and the presence (or absence) of traits that can buffer predispositions. In the study by Werner and Smith (1992), the most prominent traits that promoted resilience were an attractive personality, intelligence, persistence, a variety of interests, the capacity to be alone, and an optimistic approach to life. This study also demonstrated the interactions between the constitutional and environmental elements in resilience. Werner and Smith's cluster analysis of the protective influences operating within their cohort revealed four factors: 1) a temperament that elicited caring responses; 2) an ability to develop realistic plans, regular working habits, and skills; 3) the presence of some degree of parental support; and 4) availability of supportive adults outside the nuclear family.

Although many of the children in this study had short-term difficulties during development, resilience was the rule in the long run. Thus, whereas at adolescence two-thirds of those in the high-risk group had problems, largely with conduct disorder, when the same individuals were seen at 30 years of age, most (5/6) had become competent adults.

Clearly, resilience in children is a mixture of a good constitution and good fortune. But capacities intrinsic to the individual are also the best predictors of successful coping throughout life. Personality traits are much more useful than life events in predicting whether adults develop mental disorders.

Thus, in prospective research that followed adolescents through the life cycle (Vaillant 1977), the quality of childhood experience had little or no predictive value about the extent to which adults eventually achieved psychological maturity. Instead, school performance and defense styles were the best predictors of functioning in later life. These measures reflect the presence of adaptive personality traits.

A second element in resilience involves favorable environmental circumstances that buffer the negative effects of risks. The most important environmental element in resilience among children is the availability of social supports from the extended family, the schools, and the community (Kaufman et al. 1979; Rutter 1987a). However, the presence of favorable personality traits increases the likelihood that children at risk will actually be able to take advantage of these supports.

The mechanisms promoting resilience make good sense in an evolutionary context. If people could not bounce back from adversity, the inevitable traumas in life would interfere with fitness. In the environment of evolutionary adaptiveness (Bowlby 1969), when life may have been—in Hobbes's famous phrase—"nasty, brutish and short," traumatic events were even more common than they are now. Resilience is therefore a trait that has passed through the sieve of natural selection.

In summary, children are much tougher and more flexible than we have usually thought. This conclusion may be counterintuitive to some readers, who are accustomed to seeing early childhood as a time of great vulnerability. But that is theory. The confirming evidence is not there.

The view being taken in this book does not, of course, imply that "everything is in the genes." Constitutional factors might be compared to a landscape through which the river of life events runs. Since life is a chaotic process, the ultimate pattern resulting from this interaction is not predictable. However, the influence of life events will be influenced by the "lay of the land."

Moreover, the environment of childhood is enormously complex. Since risk factors interact with protective factors, only the most consistent effects deform personality. Circumstances can offer opportunities to reverse these effects, and there are "turning points" (Rutter 1987a) at which unexpected fortune changes the course of life's river.

Finally, there is no reason to believe that development and change end in childhood or adolescence (M. Lewis 1997). Adult developmental theory, based on long-term prospective studies (e.g., Vaillant 1977), has shown that every stage of life presents its own demands and that people continue to change in respond to these challenges. There is no reason to believe that traumatic events occurring later in life are necessarily less pathogenic than those occurring in childhood. However favorable one's childhood experiences, there is no guarantee that one will remain happy.

■ The Primacy of Early Experience: A Critique

The idea that early experiences shape personality and are strongly implicated in the development of clinical symptoms in adult life has been taken for granted by generations of therapists. The theoretical assumption is that early learning must have a greater impact than later learning, since it occurs at a time when the organism is more plastic and the child is more dependent on its parents (Millon 1969). These models also assume that the more severe the adult pathology, the earlier in childhood must be its origins (Paris 1983).

Despite their ubiquity, these ideas have not found support from empirical research. As discussed earlier, developmental psychopathology shows that, by and large, negative events occurring early in life do *not* by themselves usually lead to psychiatric disorders. Given a reasonably favorable environment, most children are resilient to stressful events. However, early stressors are often followed by later ones, so that adversities that eventually become multiple and cumulative are more likely to begin early in development (Rutter and Rutter 1993).

How can we account for the cumulative effects of stressors? One possible explanation is that when too many things go wrong, children develop a sense that life events are outside their control. This cognitive set has been termed "learned helplessness" and is theorized to be a major factor in the development of clinical depression (Seligman 1975). Another possible explanation is that continuous adversities overwhelm resilience and prevent the child from recovering from early trauma (Rutter 1987a, 1989; Rutter and Rutter 1993).

Why do so many clinicians believe that earlier events are primary? Therapists are understandably impressed by the narratives they hear from their patients. Moreover, many patients are influenced by their culture to believe that their problems must derive from childhood experiences. Therapists who also assume the primacy of early experience will be impressed by descriptions of dramatic early events, seeing them as the primary cause of patients' symptoms.

Clinical experiences often lead to incorrect conclusions about cause and effect. The problem results from drawing broad conclusions from patient samples. What practitioners may fail to take into consideration is that many individuals who have had experiences similar to those of their patients have nonetheless become well-functioning adults. Moreover, the negative effects of deprivations in *early* childhood can be counteracted by later, more positive experiences. For example, in a study of multifostered children, the effects of neglect and multiple separations proved surprisingly reversible if the children were placed in a better environment before age 7 years (Clarke and Clarke 1979).

There is another important principle to keep in mind regarding the effects of early experience. Negative events in life are not independent, but lead to each other in what has been called a "cascade." These sequences have been well described in studies of the impact of parental separation and loss on children (Amato and Booth 1997; Amato and Keith 1991; Chase-Lansdale et al. 1995; Rodgers 1994; Tennant 1988).

Although most children are able to overcome family breakdown, losing a parent leads to secondary effects. The most important of these are financial distress or depression in the custodial parent, which are risk factors in their own right. Without these cascade effects, parental separation or loss in childhood does not consistently lead to adult psychopathology.

Yet these multiple negative events, or adversities that are continuously present throughout childhood, do not always lead to serious psychopathology. Even in the face of cumulative adversities, some children have the capacity to remain resilient.

To understand the impact of negative childhood experiences on the development of mental disorders, we must make a distinction between *risk factors* and *causal explanations*. In clinical epidemiology, risk factors are most likely to be etiological when they precede the development of pathology; when they are consistently, strongly, and specifically associated with the disorder; and when there is a plausible mechanism linking the risk with the illness (Regier and Burke 1995). These criteria are rarely met in practice.

We should also keep in mind that associations between risk factors and disorders need not have *any* etiological significance. In some cases, the association can be statistically significant yet account for only a small portion of the outcome of the variance. As Kraemer et al. (1997) have recently remarked, "It is difficult to find two variables that are absolutely independent of each other. Without considering some measure of potency in the assessment, given a large enough sample size, virtually every factor could be demonstrated to be a risk factor for every outcome that follows it" (p. 339).

We must never forget that correlation need not imply causation. Associations between risks and disorders can often be accounted for by other factors, which have been termed "latent variables." Some of these latent factors involve gene–environment interactions. For example, negative experiences are more likely to occur to vulnerable children, particularly those whose problematic temperaments make it more difficult to achieve "goodness of fit" with their caregivers (Chess and Thomas 1984). Research has also shown that temperamentally difficult children are more likely to be maltreated by their parents (Rutter and Quinton 1984).

In summary, adverse life events certainly increase the likelihood—

above and beyond biological factors—of long-term psychopathological outcomes (Rutter and Maughan 1997). However, given that as many nonpatients as patients have had adverse experiences, we cannot assume a simple cause–effect relationship between life events and psychopathology.

The primacy of early experience is a hypothesis that can be discarded. It is inconsistent with a wide range of research in developmental psychology. Personal history helps us to understand some of the *mechanisms* that produce psychopathology. However, such a history is rarely by itself the primary *cause* of mental disorder.

■ The Nature of Environmental Stressors

Stressors can be specific to the individual, such as problems on the job or the breakup of a relationship. However, stressful circumstances in the wider social sphere affect virtually everyone. As we will see later in this book, social stressors are at least as important as psychological stressors in the development of mental disorders.

In Chapter 2, we reviewed the sources of the environmental contribution to personality traits and found that this component is largely "unshared." With rare exceptions, the unshared component constitutes the crucial environmental contribution to most mental disorders. Although it remains possible that this finding reflects differential parenting practices, one would still have to explain *why* parents treat their children differently, and consider whether the explanation lies in a parent's reaction to a child's temperament. For example, recent studies (Reiss et al. 1995; Pike et al. 1996) of children with conduct disorder and depression suggest that differential parenting is largely attributable to heritable characteristics in the child.

Moreover, the evidence also shows that many other life experiences, other than living with a particular set of parents, contribute to the development of personality. Despite long-standing beliefs to the contrary, the most important stressors in childhood need not necessarily arise from experiences in the family of origin. These findings are not widely known among clinicians.

There is also a very large literature showing that social and economic factors are powerful stressors that can increase the risk for mental disorders (Eaton 1986). Let us consider a few examples:

1. Long-term trends over many decades show that more people are admitted to mental hospitals when unemployment is high than when it is low (Brenner 1977).
2. Many mental disorders have strikingly different levels of prevalence at different socioeconomic levels (Eaton 1986), in different cultural settings (Murphy 1982), and in different countries (Leff 1988).
3. The prevalence of mental disorders can change rapidly over time, most probably because of changes in social structures (L. N. Robins and Regier 1991).

Social factors can also be important determinants of psychological stress. Under difficult economic conditions, more individuals become ill, generally as a result of losing a job and not being able to find another one. Even the availability of an intimate partner depends to some extent on social factors, since individuals linked to a strong social network have a better chance of finding a new person or replacing a lost person.

The impact of social factors tends to be greatest when a trait is highly prevalent. This conclusion may initially seem paradoxical. However, as we will see later in the book, many predispositions are widely distributed in the population. Thus, for each individual who develops clinical depression, bulimia nervosa, alcoholism, or attention-deficit/hyperactivity disorder, there are numerous other individuals who carry the same predisposition but do not develop the illness. By lowering the threshold of liability, social factors can change the prevalence of such disorders dramatically within a single generation, producing "cohort effects" (L. N. Robins and Regier 1991). Conversely, when predispositions are less widely distributed, or when the precipitating factors remain relatively constant from generation to generation, the prevalence of a disorder will tend to remain stable.

Interactions Between Predispositions and Stressors

Kendler and Eaves (1986) have described three mechanisms by which genes and environment interact in mental disorders. The first involves *additive* genetic and environmental effects. This is our usual way of thinking about the subject—that is, genes raise one's liability to illness to some degree, after which environmental risks further increase liability, and psychopathology develops when the total liability crosses a given threshold. A second mechanism involves genetic control of *susceptibility* to the environment. A third mechanism involves genetic control of *exposure* to the environment.

Rutter (1997) has proposed a very similar classification of gene–environment interactions: 1) passive correlations (based on parental behavior), 2) evocative correlations (in which traits elicit responses), and 3) active correlations (in which traits shape the environment).

Let us examine Kendler and Eaves' concepts in some detail. Genetic control of susceptibility to the environment means that individuals differ in the extent to which they experience life events as stressful. The same event can have totally different effects on different individuals. This applies to even the most traumatic life events.

Two mechanisms could account for these individual differences in susceptibility to stressful events. One concerns the presence of predispositions to specific symptoms. Thus, individuals who have genetic vulnerabilities to depression or anxiety will be more likely to develop these symptoms under stress than will individuals who lack such vulnerabilities. A second mechanism concerns personality traits that make individuals more vulnerable to negative events. For example, individuals who are more dependent on social approval and the support of significant others are more likely to be devastated by rejections or losses, while those who are temperamentally less responsive to the reactions of others will be less affected. For example, those who are high on the personality dimension of neuroticism (see Chapter 15) are more likely to put a pessimistic "spin" on a variety of life events.

In summary, individuals can experience the same events as negative, positive, or neutral. Therefore, we cannot assess the effects of life events without considering how they are processed (G. W. Brown and Harris 1989). The fact that the same environmental stressors produce different effects on different people is also one of the reasons for the lack of concordance in personality or psychological symptoms between siblings. Brothers and sisters who grow up in the same family and who are treated in much the same way end up being almost as different from each other as perfect strangers (Dunn and Plomin 1990; Sulloway

1996). This observation is well known to parents. It has been said that mothers with one child believe in the environment, while mothers with two children come to believe in the genes.

Genetic control of exposure to the environment means that predispositions influence both the severity and the frequency of negative life events (Kendler et al. 1993a; Thapar and McGuffin 1996). Some individuals are much more likely than others to be exposed to negative life events. To take one example, individuals with an impulsive temperament are much more likely to get into trouble with other people, which can lead to job loss and/or interpersonal rejection.

At first glance, the idea that genes influence the quality of life events might seem counterintuitive. However, on further reflection, the conclusion is perfectly logical. The explanation is that personality traits influence both exposure and susceptibility to negative environmental events.

The notion that negative events have a genetic component may be rather startling to those who assume that the environment is an external force. Yet the list of life experiences that are to some extent heritable is rather long, encompassing marital difficulties, divorce, ease in forming friendships, availability of social supports, problems at work, socioeconomic status, and educational attainment, all of which show heritabilities ranging between 30% and 50% (Kendler 1997b; Kendler et al. 1993a).

In summary, life events are *not* random or external to the individual. Although there *is* such a thing as good or bad luck in life, personality determines how likely we are to be exposed to negative events as well as our ultimate response to them. Some people suffer more than their share of life's vicissitudes. Others live "a charmed life," either because they avoid being exposed to stress or because they emerge from it relatively unscathed.

Conclusions

In summary, only the most complex relationships between multiple genetic and multiple environmental factors can account for the pathways to mental illness. The relationship between risks and disorders in psychiatry is therefore *nonlinear*.

We can be exposed to many risk factors without becoming ill. This is because personality traits, like an immune system, can either make us more vulnerable to psychopathology or protect us against mental illness (Millon and Davis 1995). However, there is always a point at which natural defenses can be overwhelmed. Mental disorders then become relatively independent of the risk factors that produced them. This is why psychopathology can emerge like ketchup does from a bottle—either not at all, or all at once.

4

The Psychoanalytic Model

Psychoanalysis is a complex set of ideas. It is a theory of how the normal human mind works. At the same time, it is a model of the origins of mental illness.

About 40 years ago, the psychoanalytic model was dominant in North American psychiatry. Although the theory has a much more restricted influence today, it retains a strong hold on the thinking of many clinicians.

The reader might reasonably feel that too much has already been written on the subject of psychoanalysis! The critics of Freud have recently had a very wide audience. K. Popper (1968) questioned the philosophical validity of a discipline whose hypotheses are often immune to disproof. Grunbaum (1984) criticized the practice of using clinical observations to prove psychoanalytic hypotheses. Gellner (1993) offered a detailed critique of the claim that the psychoanalytic method provides a privileged access to the unconscious mind. Crews (1995) and Webster (1995) have attacked both the epistemological basis of psychoanalysis and its claims to superior therapeutic efficacy.

The purpose of this chapter is not simply to add more fuel to these onslaughts. Despite all the criticisms to which it has been subjected, psychoanalysis remains a useful model for understanding how people think and feel. For this reason, it is still of value for psychotherapists, the efficacy of whose techniques depend so much on their capacity for empathy. My aim in this chapter is to address the strengths and weaknesses of the psychodynamic model as an explanation of the origins of psychopathology.

The main reason for devoting an entire chapter of this book to psychoanalysis is that, as we will see, contemporary psychodynamic models are bastions of the environmental model of mental illness. The influence of these ideas has extended far beyond the psychoanalytic movement itself. As discussed in the previous chapter, the assumption that psychopathology has its origins in early childhood experience continues to have a strong influence on the work of clinicians.

The dominance of environmentalism in contemporary psychoanalysis would probably be a great surprise to Sigmund Freud. Over time, psychoanalysis has held a rather paradoxical position in relation to the nature–nurture debate. Classical Freudian theory has often been criticized for being an *insufficiently* environmental model. Thus, many contemporary analysts, from Bowlby (1969) to Miller (1984), have taken Freud to task for placing too much emphasis on innately based fantasies while ignoring the impact of real events. Today, analysts tend to emphasize environmental trauma over factors innate to the individual.

Freud believed that intrapsychic structures, based on innate mental mechanisms, were the primary causes of the neuroses. At the same time, it was Freud (1933/1964) who first promulgated the doctrine of the primacy of early experience. This latter strain of psychoanalytic theory has continued to influence the way clinicians perceive development.

The main thrust of this chapter will be to examine how psychoanalysis became an environmental theory. Although there have been many different versions of the basic model, most theorists have assumed that both normal personality traits and psychopathology derive from experiences during childhood. As psychoanalysis has placed more and more emphasis on the child's early environment, it has evolved into a model in which genetic influences play only a minor role. In this chapter I will suggest ways in which psychodynamic theory might be modified to take into account modern knowledge about the interactions between predisposition and stress.

. . . .

How Did Psychoanalysis Become an Environmental Theory?

The Freudian Model

There were three stages in the development of the psychoanalytic model. The first two were associated with Freud, who began with an environmental bias and later focused on innate factors in development (Ellenberger 1970). In the third, post-Freudian stage, psychoanalysis again became strongly environmental.

In his initial model, Freud (1896/1962) had proposed that "hysteria" is caused by childhood sexual trauma. In his later formulations of the etiology of hysterical symptoms, Freud (1916/1963, 1933/1964) tended to explain them as rooted in Oedipal wishes. The idea that mental structures such as the Oedipus complex were innate and universal was, if anything, an anti-environmental position. However, Freud never rejected the idea that trauma could lead to psychopathology, but he continued to believe that traumatic events can be repressed and cause symptoms later in life.

As we will see in Chapter 11, the idea that repressed childhood trauma can be a major cause of adult psychopathology is alive and well among contemporary therapists (Herman 1992). As Crews (1995) has cogently pointed out, there is a direct link between Freud's ideas and the recent interest in trauma and "recovered memories" of trauma. Contemporary trauma theorists seem to perceive troubled children and adults largely as victims of the misbehavior of others. Freud (1916/ 1963), on the other hand, refused to see children as "innocent" and emphasized that they could be selfish, aggressive, or even sexually seductive.

In Freud's time, his ideas about the mind offered a useful alternative to outmoded 19th-century theories ascribing psychopathology to vague or poorly understood mechanisms involving "degeneration of the nervous system" (Hale 1995). However, in the last 25 years, Freud's concept of what is innate in mental structures has been attacked from several quarters. Feminist analysts (e.g., Sherfey 1966) have criticized Freud for basing his ideas on a crude biological determinism, as in his dictum that "anatomy is destiny," implying that the psychological differences between the sexes are rooted in anatomical differences. Other critics (e.g., Bowlby 1969; Masson 1984; Miller 1981) have argued that fantasies cannot by themselves cause pathology and that we should look for histories of real traumatic experiences in our patients. Finally, the complex theory of mental structure that Freud called "metapsychology," largely because it is incapable of being operationalized and tested, has fallen out of favor (G. Klein 1976).

Freud's biological ideas have also become anachronistic. These speculations were drawn from theories current in Freud's own time (Sulloway 1979) that have since been completely discredited and superseded. Thus, current neurobiological thinking is certainly not consistent with Freud's comparison of the mind to a complex physical mechanism in which the intrapsychic forces determining communication between the conscious and unconscious minds are like pressure gradients, and in which symptoms function like malfunctioning valves. Nor does contemporary evolutionary theory allow for any allegiance to Lamarckian mechanisms, in which characteristics acquired during the organism's lifetime can be inherited. Furthermore, modern biology has not accepted the 19th-century idea that "ontogeny recapitulates phylogeny"—that is, that the organic or psychic development of the organism recapitulates the previous course of evolution.

Since it is crucial to Freud's theory, let us focus on the construct of a biologically determined Oedipus complex. Psychoanalysis hypothesizes that oedipal feelings develop more or less independently of the environment and that they go on to have a profound influence on the psychic development of children and adults. Freud (1913/1958) even proposed that oedipal feelings developed as a result of an *event* in prehistory, the overthrow of the father by the "primal horde."

Outside psychoanalysis, such theories have met with either hostility or silence (Webster 1995). Within psychoanalysis, Freud's ideas have not been openly rejected, but rather have been either soft-pedaled or quietly shelved. Among contemporary theorists, the Oedipus complex has tended to be superseded by theories that emphasize the primacy of the bond between the child and its mother. Moreover, post-Freudian analysts have reformulated "oedipal" phenomena in a variety of other ways that give them more of an interpersonal than a structural significance (Paris 1976).

As the biological elements of psychodynamic theory have become less important, the residual environmentalist portions have become more central. In fact, the most essential aspect of contemporary psychodynamics for most therapists is probably the construct of the primacy of early experience. To review, the principles are that personality is more strongly shaped by events occurring in the earliest years of life than by those occurring later in development, and that the symptoms of mental disorders also have their roots in events during the first 5 years of life. (A critique of these positions can be found in Chapter 3.)

Freud's (1930/1961) ultimate view of human nature was dialectical: we are driven by our innate instincts, but the price of civilization is their frustration. These inescapable conflicts must inevitably cause neurosis. Freud (1908/1959) recommended, nonetheless, certain social changes, particularly a freer sexual life, which might make the human condition more bearable. In a memorable phrase, Freud (1896/1962) stated that his method of treatment was designed "to convert neurotic suffering to normal human misery."

Psychoanalysis After Freud

Not all of those who followed Freud were as pessimistic as the founder of psychoanalysis had been. If anything, the history of post-Freudian analytic practice was marked by an enormous surge of optimism. In fact, one of the reasons that defectors left psychoanalysis in its early stages was that they did not share Freud's tragic view of the human condition, but believed in the possibility of maximizing human potential, either through spiritual growth (Jung 1921) or through social change (A. Adler 1927/1978). Many of these more optimistic views were also associated with strong beliefs in the primacy of early experience. Thus, if neuroses are largely due to problems in the early years of life, therapies in which these events are uncovered might entirely reverse their effects.

In the 1930s, almost all psychoanalysts were driven out of continental Europe and had to emigrate, in most cases to either Britain or America. In Britain, psychodynamic theory moved in two opposite directions. Melanie Klein was one of the most influential psychoanalysts of her generation. Klein was a therapeutic optimist who believed that universal child analysis could prevent the development of neurosis (Grosskurth 1986). Yet she had a strong belief in innate psychic structures (M. Klein 1946) and paid even less attention than had Freud to the role of environmental stressors.

The influence of Klein's ideas continues today through the writings of analysts trained by Klein herself or by her followers. Yet the Kleinian tradition has also produced broader models of psychopathology. For example, Otto Kernberg is one of the few analytic therapists working with a predisposition–stress model. Kernberg (1975) has proposed that temperamental differences between individuals are crucial in shaping psychopathology and has hypothesized that severe personality disorders are associated with constitutionally high levels of aggression.

In contrast, the British "object relations school" (Fairbairn 1952; Guntrip 1969), although based on some of Klein's ideas, has taken a strongly environmentalist view of mental illness. Analysts of this persuasion have tended to view psychopathology as due almost exclusively to bad parenting, Some (e.g., Winnicott 1958) focused on the effects of parental neglect of a child's emotional needs, which caused the child's "true self" to be hidden behind a wall of defenses. In general, object relations theorists have been less interested in hypothesizing mental structures and more interested in the real events affecting children that interfere with the quality of their intimate relationships later in life.

Psychoanalysis in America

On the other side of the Atlantic, the psychoanalytic movement became highly influential, not only on psychiatry but on the broader intellectual culture (Crews 1986; Fancher 1995). The poet W. H. Auden (1939/1979), in an elegy on Freud's death, put it neatly: "for us, he has become, not a person, but a climate of opinion" (p. 37).

This interpenetration between psychoanalysis and American culture might help to explain some of the emphasis on the importance of the environment among contemporary psychotherapists. The cultural ideals of the United States place enormous importance on individualism, and Americans have always believed strongly in human progress (Torrey 1992). Some historians (see Hale 1995) have suggested that the roots of American culture lie in the break from Europe, the rejection of "old country" values in favor of a New World optimism, and a "can do" approach to problems in which many more things are possible than impossible. It is therefore not surprising that environmentalism has dominated the psychoanalytic movement in America.

The "neo-Freudians" (e.g., Fromm 1940/1978; Horney 1940) were transplanted European socialists whose dissent from classical analysis, and its emphasis on innate mechanisms, found support in the American intellectual climate. Like Adler, they believed that progressive political programs could change society in ways that might decrease the overall prevalence of psychopathology. Sullivan (1953) was a native-born American theorist with no clear political agenda, but his "interpersonal theory" placed much greater emphasis than did classical psychoanalysis on real—as opposed to fantasized—psychological stressors, as well as on the influence of the social environment.

Psychoanalysis has also produced a number of American "offshoots" that can no longer really be called Freudian. Several clinicians, who had been originally trained in psychoanalysis but had become disillusioned with its results, proposed entirely different modes of treatment. All of these new systems focused much more on the environmental factors in psychopathology, jettisoning Freud's intrapsychic structures in favor of more readily understood and observable constructs.

The best example of these developments is the family therapy movement (Ackerman 1966). Originating in America, family therapy moved far from its Freudian roots by conceptualizing disorders in children not as based on intrapsychic structures but rather as secondary reactions to dysfunction in the family system. (This is why family therapists usually refer to a symptomatic child as "the identified patient.") As we will see in Chapter 8, some theorists (e.g., Bateson et al. 1956) even tried to conceptualize schizophrenia as rooted in pathological family dynamics.

Currently, two of the most influential versions of psychoanalysis among practicing psychotherapists are attachment theory and self psychology. I will examine each of these in turn, demonstrating how these models have placed an environmentalist "spin" on psychoanalysis.

Attachment Theory

Of all the revisions of classical psychoanalysis, attachment theory, developed by Bowlby (1969), has made the most serious attempt to develop a model consistent with empirical research.

Although attachment theory is, historically, an offshoot of the object relations approach, it has a much broader theoretical base that attempts to integrate psychodynamics, evolutionary theory, and general systems theory. The biological grounding of the theory lies in the construct of the evolution and adaptive significance of attachment systems. Some of the major foci of psychological vulnerability in children, such as depression and anxiety, have a positive function for maintaining attachments. Nesse and Williams (1994) have made similar arguments, seeing these common psychological symptoms as exaggerations of normal reactions developed through natural selection.

Yet in most ways, attachment theory is strongly environmentalist. Bowlby (1969, 1973, 1980) accounted for many forms of psychopathology by citing deficiencies in parenting. The role of biology lay primarily in the *form* of anxious and depressive symptoms, which are genetically patterned attempts to seek proximity to a caretaker. Although Bowlby (1969) acknowledged that predispositions must play some role in psychopathology, in practice, his model takes little account of genetic factors.

The attachment literature has developed empirical evidence that parental behaviors that fail to meet biological needs for secure attachment can be pathogenic. However, the model has not properly addressed the issue of how individual differences between children influence attachment phenomena. Thus, a good deal of research (Fonagy et al. 1996; Main and Hesse 1991) has suggested that attachment styles are intergenerationally transmitted. Yet the mechanism of transmission need not be environmental, but could just as well be genetic. Moreover, with few exceptions (e.g., Thompson et al. 1988), there has been little research into genetic influences on attachment patterns that might account for the similarities in attachment styles between parents and children.

Self Psychology

Self psychology (Kohut 1970) is an even more strongly environmental variant of psychoanalysis. Although the theory has not generated much empirical research, its ideas have an obvious resemblance to attachment theory. One of the most basic assumptions is that psychic structures that develop in children are internalizations of positive or negative parental responses to their needs. The only biological element in Kohut's theory is that a child's need for parental empathy, as well as the child's need to idealize the parent, is a developmental given. The model explains the development of pathology primarily on the basis of parental behaviors such as empathic failures or traumatic disillusionments (Kohut 1977).

In summary, both attachment theory and self psychology demonstrate the extent to which environmentalism has "captured the soul" of the psychoanalytic model.

Predispositions and Psychodynamic Formulations

In the present century, we can draw a much more specific picture of the nature of genetic vulnerability than would have been possible 100 years ago. Psychoanalysts need not, therefore, continue to use outmoded cognitive models or strictly environmentalist theories of child development. It is time for contemporary psychoanalytic theory to make room in its model for the role of predispositions.

Although the basic paradigms in any science usually enjoy a long life, it is unheard of in most disciplines to quote authors whose ideas were current over a century ago. Yet this is the current condition of the psychoanalytic literature. Even when psychoanalysts move on to new formulations, they do not discard older theories.

One useful modification would be to build bridges integrating psychodynamic theory with the findings of contemporary science. In particular, psychoanalysis needs to take into account individual differences in temperament. As will be discussed in Chapter 15, these temperamental differences play a crucial role in shaping the stable characteristics of behavior, feeling, and thought that we call *personality*.

Everything that happens to us in childhood and later life is processed through our personality traits. Individual differences in personality help to explain why patients' *perceptions* of their childhood can be more important than the bare facts of experience. Spence (1983) has argued that what our patients *tell* us about their lives represents only a "narrative truth." What *actually* happened in childhood is a "historical truth" to which we ultimately have no access.

Patients and therapists may explain behaviors as the outcome of significant life events. However, like professional historians, we can rarely be sure that these narratives are accurate or that they really account for the course of events. All we have are "causal attributions," varying from highly sophisticated formulations to the commonsensical ideas embedded in "folk psychology" (Kirmayer et al. 1994b). Finally, what patients tell us about their lives inevitably mirrors our own preconceptions about which events we believe to be most significant.

Ultimately, the clinical methods of psychoanalysis can yield only narratives, not empirical data. This is why material from the therapy of patients cannot be used to reach firm conclusions about the etiology of mental disorders. Clinical evidence cannot provide data that meets the minimal standards of scientific inquiry.

In an important philosophical critique of the clinical methods used to collect psychoanalytic data, Grunbaum (1984) emphasized that what patients tell their analysts is inevitably influenced by the context of the procedure. For this reason, the information gathered in therapy does not have the same epistemological status as data obtained in other ways. In particular, perceptions, which tell us as much about the individual as about the event, provide an insufficient basis for determining whether environmental events are implicated in the etiology of a mental disorder. To establish the extent to which negative life events, either in childhood or adulthood, cause psychopathology, we need empirical investigations, preferably ones that use prospective designs.

At present, contemporary psychoanalysts are divided concerning the epistemological status of their discipline. Many analysts *are* working to integrate psychoanalysis with general psychology, and some of them are making serious attempts to develop a research base (Shapiro and Emde 1994). These recent developments within the psychoanalytic movement could eventually lead to a rapprochement between analysis and other disciplines.

We can point to several examples of this trend. D. Stern (1985) has conducted empirical studies on the nature of cognition and emotions in infants. Unlike the speculations of Melanie Klein (1946), Stern's research meets standards for scientific research. Vaillant (1977) has conducted empirical research on defense styles as predictors of psychopathology. Vaillant's studies have a sophisticated methodology, drawing on prospective samples of adolescents followed throughout their lives. Luborsky and Crits-Christoph (1990) have studied the mechanisms by which patients improve in psychodynamically oriented psychotherapy. Far from taking psychodynamic principles for granted, this research operationalizes them so that they can be measured systematically.

Over time, psychoanalysis must build more bridges of this kind. In doing so, it must be willing to put Freud's ideas to empirical tests and to discard those elements of his model that can be neither operationalized nor tested. In this scenario, psychoanalytic institutes would overcome their intellectual isolation and join the larger scientific community. Psychoanalysis is a complex amalgam of many scientific hypotheses, some of which have empirical support and others of which have been refuted (S. Fisher and Greenberg 1996; Torrey 1992). However, many of the most important ideas derived from psychoanalytic theory have never been studied empirically at all. Psychoanalysts should be collaborating with researchers in psychiatry and psychology to conduct formal research on their discipline (Kandel 1998).

Unfortunately, not all analysts are sympathetic to empiricism. Some have responded to the challenge of science not by becoming more empirical but rather by rationalizing a retreat from science. These analysts describe their methods of inquiry as "hermeneutic" (Spence 1992)—that is, concerned with the *interpretation* of ideas rather than with facts per se. In taking this stance, however, they accord the narrative elements of therapy an undeserved prestige. Moreover, this intellectual position protects theoretical formulations from having to meet the ultimate test of data collection and research methodology.

Actually, many modern psychoanalysts agree that Freud's model needs revision. Bowlby (1969) was a pioneer in the integration of psychoanalysis with biological research. More recently, Gabbard (1994) has written eloquently in defense of the psychoanalytic model, arguing that earlier criticisms have already been taken into account in modified versions of the basic theory.

The crucial limitation of psychoanalytic formulations of psychopathology remains their failure to provide an adequate account of the role of individual differences. Unique environmental events do not explain why the same events can yield entirely different outcomes. Freud once addressed this question while attempting to explain why a woman had developed a homosexual orientation. As Freud (1920/1955) himself disarmingly acknowledged,

> [s]o long as we trace the development from its final outcome backwards, the chain of events appears continuous, and we feel we have gained an insight which is completely satisfactory or even exhaustive. But if we pro-

ceed in the reverse way, if we start from the premises inferred from the analysis and try to follow these up to the final result, then we no longer get the impression of an inevitable sequence of events which could not have been otherwise determined. (p. 167)

Freud (1920/1955) also argued as follows:

Even supposing we have a complete knowledge of the etiologic factors that decide a given result, nevertheless what we know about them is only their quality, and not their relative strength. (p. 168)

Here Freud almost seems to anticipate the concept of a modern regression equation, with its weighting of multiple variables. However, even if we *could* know the relative strength of the different factors affecting development, we would still not be able to predict outcomes without considering the interactions between these factors. Moreover, a simple weighting of factors does not allow for the possibility, favored in this book, that biological variability determines predispositions, the necessary preconditions for a pathological outcome.

Without a predisposition–stress model, psychodynamic formulations become, to use a phrase from Kipling, "Just So Stories." Scientific theories need to *predict* phenomena, not just explain them in a post hoc fashion. The same psychodynamics are observable in individuals with a wide variety of psychopathologies, as well as in those with *no* significant psychopathology. Environmental events are usually triggers rather than causes of mental disorders.

Ironically, Freud, who was trained in 19th-century psychiatry, took it for granted that there were important constitutional factors in psychopathology. Thus, he assumed (Freud 1916/1963) that patients had predispositions to particular forms of psychopathology and accorded a fair degree of weight to family histories of mental illness.

Applying a predisposition–stress model would by no means eliminate the need for clinicians to understand psychodynamics in their patients. Most of us who practice psychotherapy use psychoanalytic ideas every day. These principles remain of practical use in explaining the mechanisms by which mental processes influence behavior. The problem is with the etiological aspects of the analytic model, which have become excessively environmental. As a result, psychoanalysis has fallen out of step with contemporary knowledge about the etiology of mental disorders.

A final assessment of the scientific value of psychoanalysis will be a task for the coming decades. If psychoanalysts can accept the principle that clinical observations are not the basis for empirical science, there is hope that the discipline, which has currently fallen somewhat into decline, could flourish again.

5

Nature and Nurture in the Social Sciences

In the history of ideas, phenomena rarely stand alone; rather, they are framed by a "zeitgeist." This term refers to an overall point of view shaping every field of scientific inquiry.

The nature–nurture problem is not unique to psychiatry; it has also been a crucial area of contention in the social sciences. Interactions between genes and environment not only determine the development of psychopathology but also shape variations in *normal* behavior. This chapter will attempt to place the nature–nurture problem within this broader context.

The social sciences aim to explain the structure and function of the human mind. Psychology is a basic science for all aspects of psychiatry because it studies the sources of individual differences in behavior and cognition. Sociology and anthropology are basic sciences for social and transcultural psychiatry because they describe group differences and focus on how social structures influence the way we think and the way we act.

A historical perspective is a useful way to frame the theoretical vicissitudes of the nature–nurture controversy in the social sciences. In parallel with the review of psychiatric theories presented in Chapter 1, this chapter will attempt to show how scientific ideas often reflect ideological biases.

The conflict between biological and environmental theories of the mind concerns the extent to which human nature derives from genes or experience. Ultimately, only empirical data can answer this question. But the way in which we resolve this dialectic also has political implications. If we view behavior as a "given," programmed in the genes, this could lead to a relatively conservative view of how much people can change. On the other hand, if we see behavior as largely shaped by the environment, we may take a more optimistic view of human potential and of the chances for improving human society.

In the perspective of a predisposition–stress model, both views are mistaken. Even if human behavior is shaped by genes, it is far from being fixed and immutable. However much human behavior is shaped by the environment, biology limits its variability.

The Social Sciences: A Historical Overview

The social sciences, like psychiatry, became separate disciplines only in the 19th century. Psychology arose out of philosophy and only gradually evolved into an empirical science. The most influential textbook of 100 years ago (James 1895/1981) illustrates the state of psychology during that period—an "armchair" science with little data at its disposal. Moreover, 19th-century psychology reflected the ideological biases of its time. Like psychiatry, it shared the prevailing assumption that mental mechanisms are largely innate.

In the present century, the most influential models in psychology have tended to react against past errors. Thus, the social sciences have tended to make the assumption that nurture is more important than nature in shaping human development. During the 30 years—from the 1940s to the 1970s—that environmental theories reigned in North American psychiatry, the social sciences were dominated by radical environmentalism. These models, which until recently have continued to be influential in psychology and which remain predominant in sociology and anthropology, have all assumed that behavior is a product of external forces.

As in psychiatry, these theories have been strongly challenged in recent years. A new generation of theorists have argued that behavior cannot be understood outside the context of biology, genetics, and natural selection. Tooby and Cosmides (1992) have termed previous theories the "Standard Social Science Model." The assumptions of this model can be summarized as follows:

1. Children everywhere are born with similar biological endowments and developmental potentials.
2. Individual differences among adults are due to differences in their environment.
3. The mechanisms behind these environmental factors depend on learning, either from the family or from the culture.

Let us examine the historical context of these ideas. In the first half of the 20th century, social scientists believed that there was no such thing as "human nature" (Degler 1991). Most theorists either dismissed genetic factors in behavior entirely or assumed that predisposing factors could be disregarded if they could be overridden by experience. Ultimately, in the famous phrase of John Locke (1693/1892), the infant was seen as a "blank slate" on which the environment leaves its imprint.

Environmental models in the social sciences have also been associated with an implicit political agenda. As suggested by Lewontin et al. (1985), the more we see human behavior as innate, the more we are inclined to accept existing political and social structures. On the other hand, to the extent that we see human behavior as determined by the environment, we may be more inclined to think of ways of changing that environment to improve the quality of human life.

These political implications help to explain why practicing biologists have sometimes supported environmentalist models. Stephen Jay Gould and Richard Lewontin (1979), both of whom have been sympathetic to socialism, tried to draw an intellectual line around the study of behavior. Gould, a famous exponent and interpreter of Darwinism, suggested that human behavior, unlike human anatomy and physiology, is only minimally determined by biological factors. In his view (Gould 1993), instead of containing specific behavioral programs determined by natural selection, the brain should be thought of as an all-purpose organ. The brain's capacity to make use of experience would be the only biological factor in mental development, while the development of specific thoughts, emotions, and behaviors would be accounted for by environmental input.

Environmental Models in Psychology

The Rise and Decline of Behaviorism

Behaviorism is the most radically environmental of all psychological theories. Although Pavlovian, or classical, conditioning had first been described in Russia before the First World War, behaviorism's domination of psychology was strongest in America. From the time of Watson (1926/1970) to that of Skinner (1957), behavioral psychologists influenced a generation of academics and students to believe that the genetic factors in behavior are weak and that the environment is supreme. In behaviorist theory, the brain can be thought of as a "black box," a simple telephone exchange linking stimulus and response.

Behaviorism hypothesized that if presented with the proper reinforcements, human behavior is highly malleable. The only biological factor to be considered involved innate drives, which would determine the most effective reinforcements. Above and beyond this baseline, learning principles take precedence. For example, the classic experiment of behavioral psychology involved a rat learning a task in order to obtain pellets of food. Although the rat's hunger is physiological, the behaviors used to satisfy its needs are all learned.

Dollard and Miller (1950), in a book widely influential in its time, attempted to combine behaviorist theory with psychoanalysis. These authors suggested that learning principles explain how complex human behaviors derive from biological drives. Moreover, they explicitly argued for the primacy of early experience. Another influential psychologist of the period, Clark Hull (1951/1974), thought that the entire behavioral repertoire of children could be shaped by the associations of reinforcers with simple biological needs.

Behaviorism's hold on psychology began to loosen only in the late 1950s, when empirical findings emerged that were inconsistent with its tenets. Thus, Harlow (1958) showed that attachment in infant rhesus monkeys did not depend primarily on associations with feeding but rather depended on innate needs for touch and comfort. At the same time, Chomsky (1957) showed that, contrary to Skinner's ideas (1957), learning a language cannot be explained by external reinforcements alone, but instead requires an innate capacity.

This represented a true paradigm shift, and over time, classical behaviorism was replaced with a cognitive–behavioral model. Unlike the simple stimulus–response model of behaviorism, cognitive theory is very interested in developing a model of the mind (Pinker 1997). Classical behaviorist theory had been associated with the development of classical behavior therapy, a method consistent with the assumption that there are no limits on the degree to which treatment can modify behavior. On the other hand, cognitive therapists (e.g., Beck 1986; Beck and Freeman 1990) have supported predisposition–stress models of mental disorders, and the resulting therapeutic methods set much more limited goals.

In summary, the historical evolution of psychology parallels that of psychiatry. Psychology's first models were drawn from 19th-century biology, after which the discipline was "captured" by a strongly environmentalist paradigm. More recently, with the development of behavior genetics (Plomin et al. 1990a), psychology has again become interested in genetic factors in behavior, as well as in the role of gene–environment interactions.

The IQ Controversy

Let us now examine a controversy in psychology that reflects, rather dramatically, the intensity of the nature–nurture debate.

One of the main interests of academic psychology has been the study of individual differences. Scores on intelligence tests, first developed in the early part of this century, are an important way to make these differentiations. If intelligence is inherited, then there must be some fixed quantity of cognitive capacity present at birth. Minds would be like software programs, some of which have more sophisticated designs that can deal with many different types of demands, while others are suitable only for a limited number of tasks. On the other hand, if the mind is a "blank slate," then individual differences in intellectual capacity should largely depend on external factors, such as whether one grows up in an impoverished or an enriched social environment.

The extent to which intelligence is inherited is, of course, an empirical question. Yet it has also been an emotional issue, eliciting highly political responses. Although most of the research on IQ has been carried out in America, hereditary explanations of the variance in intellectual capacity have always been controversial in the United States. Historically, IQ tests were misused to exclude immigrants with insufficient knowledge of the English language, on the rationalization that these individuals must be mentally deficient (Gould 1981). The same tests have also sometimes been used as a rationale for racial oppression. Moreover, the eugenics movement was appropriated by those who wanted to suppress reproduction in groups they disliked. In Europe, this movement led to the notorious sterilizations and exterminations of the mentally retarded by the Nazis (Kevles 1985). These historical events have influenced many to question almost any suggestion that intelligence is inherited.

Yet when we examine the empirical evidence, it is clear that IQ scores are strongly heritable, with about half of the variance attributable to genetic factors (Scarr 1981). At the same time, environmental factors are also important, in most populations influencing scores to the extent of one standard deviation (Scarr 1981). The environmental factors in intelligence include both shared and unshared components, suggesting that the family, the schools, and the community are all important in determining intellectual capacity.

Why, then, do certain scientists continue to oppose the conclusion that intellectual capacity is inherited? Their objection is that IQ itself is not a useful construct, and that "intelligence" is nothing but what intelligence tests measure. One of the most consistent criticisms of IQ testing concerns the cultural and social factors in the questions used (Gould 1981). Since test performance depends so much on vocabulary, education and social background can strongly affect IQ scores.

Another consistent objection to intelligence testing is that there is no such thing as unitary intelligence. Rather, there exists a range of capacities, with some people more intelligent in one way and others more so in other ways (Gardner 1985). Although this criticism contains a great deal of truth, scores on IQ subscales are highly intercorrelated (Scarr 1981).

Some years ago, the opponents of IQ testing had the opportunity to seize upon a juicy scandal (Lewontin et al. 1985). A British psychologist, Sir Cyril Burt, published research that seemed to show that intelligence is strongly inherited. However, it was discovered after his death that much of his data were fraudulent. (Ironically, careful behavioral genetic research in recent years shows that the contribution of the genes to intellectual capacity is at almost the same level as suggested by this imaginary data!) Burt's upper-class background fueled the arguments of those who feared that data on the heritability of intelligence could be used to suppress the less fortunate members of society. These concerns are probably justified.

One of the problems with studies of individual differences is that we can easily confuse variations between *individuals* and variations between *groups*. Individuals, whatever their race, will differ greatly in IQ, and about half of that variability is genetic. Although genetic differences between large groups are theoretically possible, they have never been demonstrated. In all probability, the most important determinants of racial differences in IQ are environmental.

The consensus among contemporary psychologists is that there are both heritable and environmental factors in intelligence, with IQ scores being determined by the interactions between these factors. The problems in sorting out the genetic and environmental factors in intelligence have a strong parallel in controversies about the roots of personality traits. This is an issue we will examine in detail in Chapter 15.

Environmental Models in Sociology

Sociology is an exception to the rule that the social sciences have been dominated at different times by theories favoring nature and nurture. By and large, sociologists have *always* been strong environmentalists.

From its inception, sociology as a discipline was dominated by a dictum proposed by the 19th-century theorist Emil Durkheim: social forces cannot be separated into component levels of analysis. As Durkheim (1951, p. 106) stated, "individual natures are merely the indeterminate material that the social factor molds and transforms." It follows that most individual differences in behavior derive from a process of social learning and not from biology.

We can place the strong environmental bias of sociological theory in historical perspective. Logically, evolution is one of the main bases for understanding social behavior. Yet Darwin never systematically applied natural selection theory to the study of social groups. A number of thinkers who followed Darwin developed a movement called "Social Darwinism," which was influential in the late 19th and early 20th century. However, their ideas were based on interpretations of evolution that have since been discarded (Cronin 1991). For example, Social Darwinists believed that evolution is progressive, that individuals act for the good of the species, and that organisms are blindly driven by "instincts." Although none of these assumptions have much scientific currency at present, they were used to justify political and social ideas in accord with a zeitgeist.

For example, many 19th-century social scientists subscribed to the theory that traditional societies were more "primitive," whereas the most modern societies represent a more advanced stage of evolution (Degler 1991). This interpretation of Darwinism was associated with strong political conservatism and provided a biological rationalization for social arrangements that in domestic politics favored the interests of the wealthy and that in international politics favored imperialism (Levins and Lewontin 1985). Today, social scientists entirely reject the construct of "social evolution." The principles of natural selection are actually much more useful in explaining why societies are *similar* than in explaining why they differ from each other.

Sociology played an important role in the rejection and overthrow of Social Darwinism. Many sociological theorists (e.g., Talcott Parsons [1967]) were interested not in changing society but rather in developing an objective and politically neutral model of social structures. However, politically oriented sociologists (e.g., Mills 1955) have used social science to criticize contemporary social arrangements. In recent decades, the field has attracted some who, like Karl Marx, believe that we should not simply accept society as it is, but instead should try to change it.

Sociology, like behavioral psychology, has downplayed its links to other disciplines, instead developing an autonomous theoretical structure of its own. This trend has been the source of many problems in the field. An analogy suggested by Tooby and Cosmides (1992) is that no biologist could afford to be ignorant of chemistry and physics. Sociology would undoubtedly benefit from theoretical models that take into consideration the innate factors on which the social environment operates.

The Sociobiology Controversy

About 20 years ago, "sociobiology" (Wilson 1975) presented a serious challenge to environmental models in sociology. Sociobiological theory applies evolutionary principles to the study of social behavior. The model created a major scientific and political controversy when Wilson suggested that sociology might become a branch of evolutionary biology, increasing the resistance of social scientists to his ideas.

Wilson's position can be briefly summarized as follows:

1. Human social behavior is genetically programmed by natural selection.
2. These programs result in a fairly universal range of social structures.
3. Since social behaviors are programmed to maximize the fitness of individuals and their relatives, altruism is usually stronger toward relatives.
4. The glue that binds nonrelated individuals to their society is "reciprocal altruism"—that is, the expectation that favors will be returned.

The critics of sociobiology pointed out a number of problems with Wilson's theory. First, we cannot make the blanket assumption that *every* form of social behavior is specifically controlled by genes. Second, as philosophers of science (e.g., Kitcher 1985) have emphasized, the theory has yet to be operationalized or put it to rigorous empirical tests. Third, some feared that Wilson was reviving Social Darwinism in a modern guise (Gould and Lewontin 1979).

The danger of biological reductionism in sociobiological theory is real. Particularly in its popularized form (e.g., Barash 1982), the model can be interpreted as suggesting the existence of genes "for" every behavior ranging from jealousy to homicide. On the other hand, the environmentalist theory that social behavior is not strongly influenced in *any* way by evolution is equally untenable. The nature–nurture debate in sociology dramatically parallels the problems facing contemporary psychiatry. Social behavior is influenced by both genes and the environment, and their interactions must be the basis for any adequate model.

Tooby and Cosmides (1992) have revived Wilson's ideas in a revised model called "evolutionary psychology." They propose replacing the Standard Social Science Model with an "Integrated Causal Model" that would link the social sciences with biology. In this view, the organism is not a passive recipient of input but rather an active force that shapes its own environment. The principles of the Integrated Causal Model can be summarized as follows:

1. The mind consists of a set of information-processing mechanisms programmed by natural selection.
2. Since these mechanisms are designed to produce behavior that solves adaptive problems, they must be structured in some detail.
3. The content of culture in all human societies reflects these mechanisms, and, although open to some modification, is fairly universal.

As a noted evolutionary theorist (T. Dobzhansky, quoted in Mayr 1982) once stated, "nothing in biology makes sense without evolution." Evolutionary social science is based on the principle that organisms need complex adaptations to survive in a complex world. Therefore, the biological universals in human nature are based on genetic "blueprints" for behavior that must be *relatively* uniform from one individual to another. Since the environment is constantly changing, some degree of variability is adaptive. However, when there is too much variation, organisms cannot survive.

Biological "givens," shaped by natural selection, determine the limits within which cultures vary. This principle can even explain *why* humans have developed cultures, which are mechanisms to reinforce the adaptiveness of social behaviors that are only partly driven by biology (Tooby and Cosmides 1992).

Evolutionary social science need not hypothesize that behaviors are hardwired in detail, only that *propensities* for certain types of behavior are built into the organism. Most of these propensities will be adaptive under a variety of environmental conditions. If they were not, they would have been selected out. This is why individuals cannot readily be conditioned to behave in ways that run counter to their biological nature: not by their parents, not by a culture, and not by totalitarian political systems.

The missing element in evolutionary social science is an adequate account of how genetic factors shape individual differences. As discussed in Chapter 2, although all mental capacities must be sufficiently adaptive to pass through the sieve of natural selection, there need not be only *one* form of adaptation that promotes fitness. Rather, humans have a range of adaptive designs, each of which, depending on the environment, can be functional. These are the differences that help account for differential vulnerabilities to illness.

Environmental Models in Anthropology

Anthropology as a discipline has always had dual roots, as reflected by its cultural and physical branches. This may help explain why the field has been rather more open than has sociology to examining the interfaces between biology and culture. Mead (1950/1975) took the position that social behavior always has genetic components. Prominent anthropologists (D. E. Brown 1991; Murdock 1975) have documented universal behavioral characteristics found in all cultures. Many anthropological theorists (e.g., Levi-Strauss 1969) have also been "structuralists" who aimed to identify the innate rules that all cultures follow. For example, Harris (1979) has advocated a biologically based theory termed "cultural materialism." Moreover, some contemporary anthropologists (e.g., H. E. Fisher 1992; Fox 1993; Tiger 1969; Wright 1994) have strongly rejected the assumptions of environmental models, instead openly embracing evolutionary models.

Yet the dominant interest in the history of anthropology as a discipline remains the study of cultural differences. The most basic theoretical principle of cultural anthropology has been *cultural relativism* (Geertz 1983). This construct implies that although there are many variations in human social behavior, there are few "universals." Therefore, a very wide range of cultural arrangements can be found in different societies.

Cultural relativism has many political implications. By studying cultural variations, anthropologists can show that there is no one "right" way of organizing a society, a point of view particularly welcome in democratic political systems. Generations of university students taking introductory courses in anthropology have been taught that human nature is almost infinitely malleable. The principle is often illustrated by anecdotes describing unusual patterns of behavior in unfamiliar cultures. The moral of these stories is clear: however much we take our own culture for granted, it is only one of many possible ways to structure a society. What is not always consistently taught, however well documented in the anthropological literature (Murdock 1975), is that universal patterns of behavior exist in *all* cultures.

The biases of cultural anthropology can be better understood in historical context. In the 19th century, reflecting the beliefs of the time, anthropologists (e.g., Tylor 1895/1964) thought that European civilization represented the highest stage of human evolution and that cultures in less developed countries were "primitive" antecedents of civilization. Darwin himself had believed in these ideas (Gould 1993). The pioneers of cultural relativism in contemporary anthropology (Benedict 1934/1961; Boas 1938; Mead 1926/1971) sought to remedy this error. They assumed that no one cultural form was necessarily more adaptive than any other. Moreover, they agreed with Durkheim (1951) that social forces shape behavior like clay.

Cultural anthropologists are often highly sympathetic to the societies they study. One sometimes has the impression that they are telling us that modernity has lost something important that is retained in traditional cultures. Since the time of Jean-Jacques Rousseau, many intellectuals have believed in a "myth of the noble savage," imagining that humanity was happier in a "state of nature" before being corrupted by civilization.

Freeman (1983) has helped to put these biases into a historical perspective. He documented how the pioneer anthropologist Franz Boas sent his student Margaret Mead to Samoa, with the overt aim of proving that the sexual problems of North American adolescents were absent in the South Seas. Mead (1926/1971) dutifully but inaccurately went on to claim in a best-selling book that Samoans lived in a sexual paradise of "free love." Freeman, an expert on Samoa, showed that the Samoans are not an unusually happy people and never have been, and that they have as many sexual problems as Americans. This story demonstrates that, like the psychoanalytic methods criticized by Grunbaum (1984), anthropological observations are subject to systematic biases that need to be tested with quantitative research methods.

Mead had helped promulgate the idea that people are happy and innocent in traditional societies. This belief has always had a romantic appeal. It is reminiscent in many ways of the common idea that *children* are born innocent but are eventually corrupted by their parents and by society. Both of these myths might be thought of as contemporary versions of Genesis, marked by an expulsion from Eden, leaving behind memories of a lost paradise. This version of the biblical myth of "man's fall" implies that children are naturally good—until their parents make them bad.

Summary

The dialectic between nature and nurture is an issue for all students of human behavior. Although biological thinking in psychiatry and the social sciences is experiencing a major revival, it need not take the simplistic form it had in the 19th century. A more sophisticated view of genetic mechanisms could help reduce intellectual resistance to the importance of biology in human behavior.

In the long run, historians will likely judge that the radical environmentalism of the 20th century has run its course. This model may be thought of as a product of a specific moment in human history, when the rapid social changes producing modernity made it seem as if the very idea of human nature was an illusion, and that behavior could take almost any imaginable form.

A more balanced reading of the scientific evidence would lead to the conclusion that although biology does not determine how we live our lives, it does define the *constraints* on human possibilities (Konner 1983). Genes establish the limits within which the environment has its effects and within which we can develop our individual potential.

6

Predisposition and Stress in Medical Illness

The same mechanisms that determine the etiology of mental disorders also apply to medical illnesses. In the future, psychiatry will probably look much more like internal medicine than it does today. It is therefore useful to frame psychiatric illness in the larger context of medical research.

This chapter will describe a group of chronic medical diseases that emerge from interactions between genetic and environmental factors. These pathways to illness make sense only in the light of a stress–diathesis model. Readers with a background in the health sciences may already be familiar with some of these findings.

I will first examine the implications of polygenic mechanisms of inheritance in chronic diseases. I then review evidence for genetic effects on longevity. One chronic illness—coronary artery disease—will be described in greater detail. I conclude the chapter with a brief review of the gene–environment interactions in essential hypertension, diabetes mellitus, bronchial asthma, peptic ulcer, and cancer.

Much of the information in this chapter depends on research methods described in Chapter 2. The increasing number of large-scale twin registers that exist in North American and Europe have helped investigators to make significant advances in determining the degree to which chronic diseases are heritable. However, obtaining this information is only the first step toward the ultimate goal of understanding the precise genetic mechanisms involved in predispositions to these diseases. Unraveling these mechanisms will probably require further advances, primarily through genetic linkage methods.

Polygenic Inheritance and Chronic Diseases

Historically, medical genetics focused on relatively rare conditions transmitted via classical Mendelian inheritance. More recently, the cutting edge of research has involved identifying gene loci associated with diseases with more complex genetic patterns. The methods involve gene linkage studies, often using histocompatibility antigens as markers for gene loci (J. L. Goldstein 1994). Because of recent breakthroughs in these techniques, researchers can now actively seek specific gene loci related to specific diseases. When we can identify several such loci, each of which accounts for part of the variance in the development of a particular illness, we are on the way to developing a useful model of complex traits.

A large body of evidence supports the principle that genetic susceptibility to common chronic diseases involves polygenic mechanisms of inheritance (Bell 1993; J. L Goldstein 1994; Summers 1993). The most important of these common illnesses are coronary artery disease, essential hypertension, diabetes mellitus, peptic ulcer, and schizophrenia, but similar mechanisms apply to many other conditions.

When phenotypes depend on interactions between multiple loci, some genes will increase the risk for illness, while other genes will reduce the risk. Depending on both genetic and environmental factors, overall liability can cross a threshold that determines whether overt disease develops and how severe that disease is.

Genetic susceptibility is therefore a *necessary* condition for the development of most chronic diseases; such susceptibility determines which type of illness the individual can develop. It is not, however, a *sufficient* condition for most diseases, which will become clinically apparent only when environmental factors increase liability beyond a certain threshold. As we will see later in this book, this principle applies to most mental disorders.

Just as predispositions are polygenic, stressors are polyenvironmental. To quote a researcher in cardiac disease (R. R. Williams 1988), "most major chronic diseases probably result from the accumulation of environmental factors over time in genetically susceptible persons." Natural selection leads organisms to evolve mechanisms of resistance against disease, so that only the cumulative effects of multiple environmental insults will overwhelm these defenses. As discussed in Chapter 3, the same principle explains the cumulative effects of psychosocial adversities.

Chronic medical diseases, like mental disorders, are heterogeneous in etiology (Stehbens 1985). In different individuals, the same illness may reflect different genetic and environmental components. As discussed in Chapter 2, different levels of genetic susceptibility often lead to multiple thresholds of liability for the development of a disease. When genetic factors are stronger, illness tends to develop at an earlier age. When diseases have an early onset, there has not been time for environmental risks to accumulate and to provoke the onset of illness. Early-onset diseases are therefore more likely to be associated with a stronger genetic loading. Conversely, a disease that develops later in life is more likely to involve relatively weaker genetic factors but stronger environmental factors. The older the person is, the longer the time available for environmental stressors to exert their cumulative effects.

Genetic and Environmental Factors in Longevity

When we apply for life insurance, the insurance company conducts a serious and anxiety-provoking series of investigations to assess our medical status. The insurer tends to focus on a few basic issues: whether we can pass a physical exam and whether common markers of vulnerability to illness, such as glucose levels and blood pressure, are within normal limits. Before being examined, we are required to answer a list of questions on the insurance form. The most important item on the questionnaire concerns the longevity of our parents. From large actuarial data banks on survival, insurers know that, on the average, they can make more money on those of us who have long-lived parents, and they are more likely to lose money on those of us whose parents have had the misfortune to die young.

Premature death is strongly influenced by genetic factors. Early death has many different causes, each of which has its own heritable component. Therefore, twin or adoption methods can be used to study the phenomenon of longevity as a whole.

Sorensen et al. (1988) studied a cohort of Danish adoptees and compared their longevity with that of their adoptive and biological parents. Using model-fitting analyses to estimate genetic and environmental factors affecting outcome, they found that death occurring *before* the age of 60 depends strongly on inheritance. The explanation is that most of the diseases that reduce longevity have a large heritable component. On the other hand, death *after* the age of 60 was much more strongly related to environmental factors.

It has not always been true that a short life span depends on genetic vulnerability. Today most people live out a full life span and die of the diseases of old age: myocardial infarction, stroke, or cancer. Yet until quite recently, infectious diseases were the major cause of premature death. In spite of the acquired immunodeficiency syndrome (AIDS) epidemic, mortality from infection among young people has never been lower than it is today.

Genetic factors play some role in the liability to infectious diseases, by influencing the strength of immunity to specific infectious agents (Childs et al. 1992). For example, heredity is one factor that determines whether an individual is likely to develop tuberculosis (Rumantsyev 1992), and at least one gene responsible for the vulnerability to this disease has been mapped, cloned, and sequenced. More recently, it has been shown that about 10% of the North American population has a genetic resistance to developing human immunodeficiency virus (HIV) infection (Dean et al. 1996). However, the heritable factors operating in infectious diseases are generally much weaker than those in the diseases of old age.

Research is now identifying the hereditary predispositions to chronic diseases with more and more precision. Biological markers, such as histocompatibility antigens, that reflect immunological differences, are being used by researchers and clinicians to determine specific vulnerabilities in each individual (Faraone and Tsuang 1995). With time, all of us will no doubt receive a gene profile telling us which diseases we are most prone to develop. Although some individuals might respond to this information with anxiety, such profiles should be useful for most people as a guide to prevention strategies. We would need to research the question of whether people in the possession of such information would actually change their habits. They would at least have knowledge about which kinds of environmental stressors they should go out of their way to avoid.

We will now review research on predisposition and stress in specific illnesses. (These findings are summarized in Table 1.)

TABLE 1. Evidence for genetic and environmental factors in chronic medical diseases

Disease	Evidence for genetic predispositions	Precipitating environmental stressors
Coronary artery disease	MZ-DZ differences	Diet, smoking, psychosocial factors
Diabetes mellitus	MZ-DZ differences	Unknown in type I; diet in type II
Essential hypertension	MZ-DZ differences	Diet, alcohol, psychosocial factors
Bronchial asthma	MZ-DZ differences	Antigen exposure
Peptic ulcer	Positive family history	Diet, infection
Cancer	Mutations in oncogenes; mutations in tumor suppressors	Smoking, diet, exposure to toxins

Note. DZ = dizygotic twins; MZ = monozygotic twins.

Coronary Artery Disease

Coronary artery disease leading to myocardial infarction is the leading cause of death in industrialized countries (Bierman 1994). It is therefore not surprising that this condition has been the subject of an enormous amount of research. Since we have a fair amount of data about the disease's heritability, and since the environmental factors operative in coronary artery disease are better understood than those in most other chronic diseases, it provides us with an excellent example of the interactions between predispositions and stressors.

Family history studies (Hopkins et al. 1986) as well as twin studies (Motulsky and Brunzell 1992) demonstrate a genetic component in coronary artery disease. This predisposition is multifactorial. There might be a specific genetic factor creating a vulnerability to arteriosclerosis in the coronary arteries. Alternatively, the heritability of coronary artery disease could reflect its association with other genetically influenced conditions that are themselves risk factors for coronary artery disease: obesity, hypertension, and non–insulin-dependent diabetes mellitus (Austin 1993; Slyper and Schechtman 1994). There are also less common conditions of strongly genetic origin that carry a particularly high risk for atherosclerosis, most particularly hyperlipidemia (Bierman 1994).

A recent twin study of American veterans of the Second World War (Carmelli et al. 1994b) found little difference between monozygotic (MZ) and dizygotic (DZ) concordances for coronary artery disease in the population as a whole. However, when the researchers examined the severity of disease, there were strong genetic effects at both extremes of the distribution, with significant heritability for coronary artery disease observed both in subpopulations with severe ischemia and in those with an unusually low prevalence of heart disease.

In a large-scale twin study conducted in Sweden, Marenberg et al. (1994) found substantial MZ–DZ differences for early death from coronary artery disease. Summarizing their results, they stated: "our findings suggest that at younger ages, death from coronary heart disease is influenced by genetic factors in both women and men. The results also imply that the genetic effect decreases at older ages." Thus, findings from several studies of coronary artery disease confirm the principles discussed in Chapter 2, in that groups with greater genetic vulnerability tend to have more severe disease as well as an earlier onset of disease.

The major focus of research on coronary artery disease has been on the disease's environmental risk factors (Dawber 1980). Striking increases in the prevalence of coronary artery disease over time (Feinlieb 1984) support the importance of environmental factors in its etiology. Of course, all of the diseases of old age are attaining higher prevalence with the increased longevity of the general population. However, studies of the environmental factors in coronary artery disease indicate that many of these risk factors are becoming more prevalent, making coronary artery disease more common.

The importance of diet in coronary artery disease was shown many years ago in a study comparing the disease's prevalence among Japanese immigrants in Hawaii with that among Japanese who had remained in their homeland (Keys et al. 1966). Whereas those living in Japan had a rather low rate of coronary artery disease, immigrants had the same rate as other Americans. One of the most likely explanations for the difference in prevalence is that the immigrants replaced their low-fat Japanese diet with typical American high-fat meals.

Many other studies have documented the link between diet and atherosclerosis (Bierman 1994). These findings have led the general public to be seriously concerned about levels of fat in the diet. What is not always understood is that there are important interactions between diet and genetic susceptibility. It is those individuals with a genetic susceptibility to coronary artery disease who need to be particularly careful about what they eat. The other major environmental factor associated with coronary artery disease is cigarette smoking (Feinlieb 1984). There is no controversy about the increased risk associated with this factor, although some smokers are more affected than others.

In contrast, the role of personality factors in coronary artery disease—specifically, of the "type A" personality (Friedman 1969)—continues to be debated. The current consensus is that only one component of type A personality, a high level of hostility, constitutes an independent risk factor for the disease (M. G. Goldstein and Niaura 1992). Nor have behavioral genetic studies shown that type A personality in itself constitutes a heritable personality dimension (Tambs et al. 1992).

Psychosocial factors are more strongly related to coronary artery disease mortality than to its overall etiology. These include general risk factors for any medical disease: being single, having few social supports, and lacking money (R. B. Williams et al. 1992). There is also evidence that comorbid major depression predicts death from cardiac disease (Carney et al. 1988).

One might be tempted to conclude that those fortunate individuals who have no genetic vulnerability to atherosclerosis can eat what they like and smoke as much as they wish. However, no one is really *that* lucky! Many of the same environmental risk factors—diet, smoking, stress—are associated with the other major causes of mortality from other chronic diseases, including cancer.

In summary, a strong genetic vulnerability, either to atherosclerosis itself or to comorbid illnesses, is associated with premature cardiac death. Cardiac illness in old age is associated with a weaker genetic predisposition and a stronger influence of environmental risk factors, both biological and psychosocial.

Because we know so much about it, coronary artery disease provides, in many ways, a good model for elucidating the etiological mechanisms of mental disorders. The factors influencing biological vulnerability to the disease are complex. The environmental factors leading to this illness are also multiple. In most people, coronary artery disease develops from a combination of many risk factors, both genetic and environmental.

I will now review, in less detail, how this same model applies to a variety of other chronic diseases in medicine.

Applications to Other Chronic Diseases

Diabetes Mellitus

Diabetes mellitus has two distinct forms: insulin-dependent diabetes mellitus, or type I, and non–insulin-dependent diabetes mellitus, or type II. The predispositions to these two types may be independent, since histocompatibility markers suggest that type I cases are associated with at least one gene locus on chromosome 6, while no association is apparent for type II cases (Foster 1994).

Both type I and type II diabetes are strongly genetic (Matsuda and Kuzuya 1994; Rotter et al. 1992a). In type I, two major genes have been localized to the human leukocyte antigen (HLA) complex on chromosome 6. Susceptibility is highest when both are present, but only a third of those with the predisposition will develop the disease (Rotter et al. 1992a). Kumar et al. (1993) found that greater levels of heritability are associated with an earlier age at onset of the type I form. In type II, family history studies (Foster 1994) and twin studies have confirmed a large genetic component, with unusually high levels of concordance among MZ twins (Rotter et al. 1992a).

The two types of diabetes mellitus are triggered by different environmental factors. Although we do not know the precise mechanism involved in type I, some theories implicate either viral infection of pancreatic beta cells or an autoimmune process that destroys these cells (Field 1988; Foster 1994). In type II diabetes, diet is a particularly crucial factor.

It is also instructive to note that the liability to type II diabetes mellitus overlaps with vulnerabilities for related illnesses. Carmelli et al. (1994a) compared MZ and DZ concordances for the joint occurrences of hypertension and type II diabetes, hypertension and obesity, and type II diabetes and obesity. In each case, the MZ concordances were above 30%, as compared with DZ concordances of 3% to 15%. Multivariate modeling of the data suggested that a common latent factor mediates the clustering of hypertension, diabetes, and obesity. This common factor showed both genetic (59%) and environmental (41%) effects.

These genetic overlaps have consequences for environmental risks. Obesity itself involves a fairly strong genetic component (Bray 1992). Because these two vulnerabilities covary, it can be more difficult for individuals with type II diabetes to lose weight.

Essential Hypertension

The predisposition to hypertension is a necessary condition for the development of this disease (Burke and Motulsky 1992). Genetic factors have been estimated to account for 20% of the variance in the risk for hypertension (G. H. Williams 1994). The most recent twin study conducted to date (Carmelli et al. 1994c) found strong genetic factors in the disease, with an MZ concordance of 62% and a DZ concordance of 36%. In a long-term prospective study, Vaillant and Gerber (1996) found that a pyknic body build (characterized by short stature, broad girth, and powerful muscularity)—a genetically determined trait—predicted the later development of hypertension.

However, even in the presence of this predisposition, individuals may never become hypertensive unless stressed by the environment. Such stressors include excessive salt in the diet, obesity, and high alcohol consumption, as well as psychosocial factors such as large family size and crowding (G. H. Williams 1994). This finding was recently confirmed by Carmelli et al. (1994c), who reported that weight gain, alcohol, and exercise are all related to the development of hypertensive disease.

The other side of this coin is that environmental stressors need not cause hypertension in the absence of a predisposition. In a recent study (Midgley et al. 1996), high salt intake was not a risk factor for hypertension in normotensive populations. This implies that people need to know their predispositions before deciding which stressors to avoid.

Bronchial Asthma

Since bronchial asthma is heterogeneous and has a very high prevalence (McFadden 1987), genetic factors are somewhat difficult to measure in this disease. Twin studies have shown that bronchial reactivity to allergens is heritable (Meyers and Marsh 1992). Several other lines of evidence point to the existence of a predisposition to bronchial asthma (Knapp and Mathe 1985). Sarafino and Goldfedder (1995) found large MZ–DZ differences in concordance for the disease (59% versus 24%) as well as for disease severity. In a population-based Finnish twin study, Nieminen et al. (1991) also found MZ–DZ differences in disease concordance and severity, with a heritability of 36%.

These genetic vulnerabilities are insufficient in themselves to cause bronchial asthma. Interactions between genetic predispositions and environmental stressors, such as antigens, are necessary for the threshold of liability for this disease to be crossed.

Peptic Ulcer

Although peptic ulcer disease is heterogeneous, most studies suggest that it is heritable (Rotter et al. 1992b). The evidence derives largely from family history studies (McGuigan 1994). The genetic predisposition to peptic ulcer might be associated with excessive gastric acidity and/or abnormal gastrin secretion (Mirsky 1958). There is also a weak association between duodenal ulcer and a biological marker, group O blood (McGuigan 1994).

Although individuals will develop peptic ulcer only if they have a specific predisposition to the disease, environmental factors are necessary conditions. Most recently, an infectious bacterial agent, *Helicobacter pylori,* has been implicated in the pathogenesis of ulcers (Peterson 1991). Additional environmental risk factors derive from diet and smoking. Despite much theoretical speculation on the subject, there does not appear to be any specific psychological profile characteristic of peptic ulcer patients (McGuigan 1994).

Cancer

Some types of cancer are strongly heritable, while other types depend more on exposure to environmental stressors. Many neoplasms, such as breast cancer, have both heritable and nonheritable forms.

Pathological changes in cellular DNA are associated with genetic predispositions to cancer. Cell growth is determined by the balance between two genetic systems: proto-oncogenes and tumor suppressor genes (Weinberg 1996). Mutations in the proto-oncogene system can produce oncogenes that promote cancer. Mutations in the tumor suppressor system can interfere with the backup system that eliminates cancer cells by signaling them to die (Raff 1996).

Both of these genetic systems are heritable, and both therefore account, at least in part, for genetic predispositions to cancer. Alternatively, environmental factors can cause "somatic mutations" that produce the same effects as genetic factors. Mutations in *p53,* a specific tumor suppressor gene, are seen in about half of all cancer patients (Raff 1996).

Cancer may occur as a result of a "two-hit model" (Knudson 1996). According to this mechanism, separate mutations—one genetically associated and one environmentally precipitated—in at least two genes would be required for cancer to occur. For example, some types of breast cancer are associated with heritable tumor suppressor genes (BRCA-1 and BRCA-2) that can be activated by a variety of pathogenic factors. Thus, environmental factors, such as smoking, diet, or exposure to toxins, can also activate oncogenes. However, genes control the threshold at which these factors can cause mutations and determine environmental sensitivity to carcinogens in the environment.

There is strong empirical evidence for these genetic factors in cancer.

It has long been known that several types of malignant neoplasms run in families (Littlefield 1984). Although twin studies of the vulnerability to cancer have been rather uncommon, in one recent large-scale study (Braun et al. 1994a), MZ twins had a significantly higher concordance than DZ twins for death from all forms of cancer. Moreover, in accord with the principles discussed in Chapter 3, cancers with an early onset are more strongly genetic than those with a later onset (Weinberg 1996).

The strength of the predispositions to cancer depends on the type of neoplasm, and it should not be assumed that all malignancies involve equivalent genetic factors. Let us consider two examples. For prostate cancer, a large Swedish twin study (Gronberg et al. 1994) found substantial differences in concordance between monozygotes and dizygotes. On the other hand, for lung cancer, studies of a very large twin registry found no differences between MZ and DZ twins in concordance (Braun et al. 1994b). The findings of the latter study were particularly interesting in that smoking showed a heritable component, while lung cancer did not. This example shows that the genetic vulnerability to disease may depend on an intermediate mechanism. In this case, personality traits of impulsivity, leading to smoking, determined exposure to the environmental factors that place individuals at risk of developing lung cancer.

In summary, although strong predispositions are involved in many types of cancer, many forms are preventable, since the environmental factors that uncover these predispositions can often be avoided or ameliorated.

Conclusions

Research into the interaction between predisposition and stress in human disease is still in its early stages. However, a general pattern emerges from the findings reviewed here. Most chronic medical illnesses demonstrate some degree of genetic vulnerability, but overt illness does not develop unless precipitated by environmental stressors. This model can also be applied to the major disorders in psychiatry.

PART II

. . . .

Mental Disorders

7

Disorders, Diagnoses, and Traits

To assess the role of nature and nurture in mental disorders, we need to know whether the diagnostic entities we are studying are actually valid. Therefore, before embarking on a survey of the literature on predisposition and stress in specific disorders, we must address the following problems:

1. The limitations in the present classification system of mental disorders
2. The criteria used to determine whether diagnostic categories are valid
3. The relationship between traits and disorders

What Is A Mental Disorder?—The Limits of the Diagnostic and Statistical Manual (DSM)

The categorization of medical illnesses changes fairly slowly. Although physicians who attended medical school 30 years ago will find a great deal of previously unknown information in contemporary medical texts, the names of diseases will, in most cases, be the same.

In contrast, the classification of psychiatric disorders has changed dramatically over time. The main reason this is so is that mental disorders are defined on the basis of phenomenology rather than etiology. We still know too little about the causes of psychiatric illness to develop an etiologically based system. Thus, it was a wise decision to replace the earlier DSM classifications, which were often based on dubious causal models, with the relatively atheoretical schemata of DSM-III (American Psychiatric Association 1980) and DSM-IV (American Psychiatric Association 1994).

Ultimately, however, most of the present categories of mental disorder will have to be replaced. Future editions of the DSM will probably use a schema rooted in an understanding of genetic predispositions. When we know the biological mechanisms involved in psychopathology, psychiatric diagnoses will look very different from those we use today.

One of the inevitable consequences of the present classification is that the boundaries around categories are fuzzy (Tucker 1998). In fact, most of the DSM diagnoses describe fairly heterogeneous populations of patients. As a result, categories overlap with each other, and most patients require multiple diagnoses to account for their symptoms. The high levels of comorbidity in clinical populations are nothing but an artifact of our diagnostic system (Jensen and Hoagwood 1997).

Yet the decision to encourage multiple diagnoses in DSM was also rational. We usually lack enough information to determine whether any diagnosis is primary or secondary. We do not know, for example, whether depression or anxiety disorders are separate entities (Judd and Burrows 1992). We do not know whether bipolar and unipolar depression are separate diseases (Gershon 1990). We do not even know whether schizophrenia and bipolar disorder are truly distinct entities (Kendell 1974).

The comorbidity promoted by the DSM system is, however, a serious problem for psychiatric research. Multiple diagnoses are particularly common in the patients we most need to study—those with the most severe levels of dysfunction (Kessler et al. 1994). We have to cope with a system that promotes fragmentary categories and that is unable to provide superordinate diagnostic categories that would account for multiple sectors of dysfunction.

In spite of these problems, any overall assessment of the value of

DSM must be, in balance, positive. The situation parallels an old saw about democracy: it is the worst possible system—with the exception of any conceivable alternative! Even if DSM fails to reflect a coherent etiological model for understanding psychopathology, it provides us with an essential common language for clinical practice and research. Therefore, the rest of this book will, with minor exceptions, follow the standard DSM classification of mental disorders.

Determining Diagnostic Validity

Senior psychiatrists can hardly be blamed for some degree of skepticism about the longevity of the current diagnostic categories. In my own case, I learned DSM-I (American Psychiatric Association 1952) as a medical student, DSM-II (American Psychiatric Association 1968) as a resident, and DSM-III after 8 years of practice. I can only be grateful for the conservative spirit that guided the revision process that led to DSM-IV.

Thirty years ago, the validity of psychiatric diagnosis was under attack from a variety of directions. Some psychoanalysts (e.g., Menninger 1963) have argued that all psychopathology lies on a continuum, and that any categorization obscures the underlying dynamics of mental illness. Psychologists (e.g., Eysenck 1973) have pointed out that psychiatrists cannot agree on their own diagnoses and have suggested that categories could usefully be replaced by scores on underlying trait dimensions. Sociologists (e.g., Scheff 1975) have argued that diagnoses are nothing but "labels" that stigmatize patients.

To its credit, psychiatry has responded constructively to all these criticisms. The research that will be quoted in this book, by demonstrating the biological roots of psychiatric disorders, shows that mental illness is most certainly not a myth. When studies showed that psychiatrists in America and Britain could not agree whether their patients had schizophrenia or bipolar disorder (Cooper et al. 1972), diagnostic criteria were developed to ensure that American and British diagnoses would be concordant in the future. (Essentially, the Americans ended up agreeing that the British had been right!) The development of DSM-III, and the adoption of this system in most parts of the world, became possible only because psychiatrists frankly admitted the inadequacies of their previous classifications.

In America, diagnostic reform emerged out of the work of a group of psychiatrists at Washington University in St. Louis who were responsible for the Research Diagnostic Criteria (Feighner et al. 1972), which was a kernel for the later development of DSM-III. Two leaders of this group, E. Robins and Guze (1970), described five basic criteria for the validity of any psychiatric diagnosis: 1) precise clinical description, 2) laboratory studies identifying biological markers, 3) clear delimitation from other disorders, 4) a characteristic outcome in follow-up studies, and 5) a genetic pattern in family history studies.

The Robins and Guze criteria are not a standard that can be met at present, but rather a blueprint for the future. With the possible exception of certain brain disorders, none of the major psychiatric disorders meets all of these criteria. However, some criteria have been met for some disorders. Thus, precise clinical description is the basis of the DSM system, with its specific criteria sets for each diagnosis. The criteria for schizophrenia make a serious attempt to separate this disorder from other psychoses. However, most of the diagnoses in the DSM seriously overlap with each other. Some disorders, such as schizophrenia, have a characteristic outcome. Most do not. Some disorders, such as bipolar illness, demonstrate a clear genetic pattern in family history studies. Most seem to be biologically heterogeneous. Hardly any diagnoses are consistently associated with specific biological markers.

Nonetheless, most of the present psychiatric diagnoses remain *clinically* useful, in that they describe entities that most practitioners recognize and can agree on, thus providing tools for communication between clinicians. A great deal of useful findings have emerged from studies using the DSM classification. Ultimately, this is the research that will be used to create a new and better system.

Traits, Disorders, and Adaptation

Many of the problems in the present diagnostic system become clearer in the light of a predisposition–stress model. If there is continuous variation between normality and pathology, it should not really be surprising that we have difficulty classifying mental disorders into discrete entities. If categories are not "real" entities, we should expect to find sharp boundaries between them (Claridge 1985). Instead, a large number of mental disorders can be understood as extreme points on a continuum between normality and pathology.

What is inherited when there is a genetic vulnerability to psycho-pathology? Most mental disorders have a large genetic component, and the more severe disorders are likely to be more heritable. As discussed in Chapter 2, when we think in terms of natural selection, it seems to make no sense at all for *any* mental illness to be inherited! The only way to make sense of this paradox is to assume that what is genetically trans-mitted is usually a *trait*. In other words, individual differences are shaped by genes, which produce characteristics that can be adaptive under one set of circumstances and maladaptive under another set. This helps to explain why, even in the presence of predispositions, heritability need not be expressed unless environmental stressors are present.

This model is compatible with the hypothesis that mental disorders reflect aberrations in hardwired evolutionary programs. Chapter 5 de-scribed the application of evolutionary principles to the social sciences. "Evolutionary psychiatry" is a parallel development.

Three recent books (McGuire and Trossi 1996; Nesse and Williams 1994; Stevens and Price 1996) have outlined a Darwinian approach to the etiology of mental disorders. The essential idea behind these models is that most mental disorders are maladaptive variants of adaptive mechanisms. This principle cannot, however, be applied universally. In some cases, mental disorders demonstrate sharp qualitative breaks from normality (as is the case for certain brain disorders).

Summary

The discussion in this chapter serves as a introduction to Part II of this book. For the convenience of the reader, the most important findings to be reviewed in forthcoming chapters are summarized in Table 2.

The range of mental disorders that can be understood as exaggera-tions of normal trait variations is wide. In later chapters, we will see that depressive illness, anxiety disorders, personality disorders, substance use disorders, eating disorders, attention-deficit/hyperactivity disorder, and conduct disorder all lie on a continuum between normality and pa-thology. In the chapter on schizophrenia, we will suggest that even the most severe forms of mental disorder can be understood as pathological exaggerations of normal variations. In the light of evolutionary theory, psychopathology appears to be normality gone awry.

TABLE 2. Evidence for genetic and environmental factors in mental disorders

Disorder	Evidence for genetic predispositions	Precipitating environmental stressors
Schizophrenia	Twin studies, adoption studies, family studies	?Neurodevelopmental
Bipolar mood disorder	Twin studies, family studies	Unknown
Unipolar mood disorder	Twin studies, family studies	Life events
Panic disorder	Twin studies, family studies	Life events
Generalized anxiety disorder	Twin studies	Unknown
Posttraumatic stress disorder	Twin studies, family studies	Traumatic events
Alcoholism	Twin studies, adoption studies, family studies	Availability, social approval
Anorexia nervosa	Twin studies, family studies	Cultural factors
Bulimia nervosa	Inconclusive	Cultural factors
Attention-deficit/ hyperactivity disorder	Twin studies, adoption studies, family studies	Expectations at school
Conduct disorder	Inconclusive	Family dysfunction
Personality disorders	Twin studies show trait heritability	Family dysfunction

8

Schizophrenia

▮ The Battleground

Clinicians today take it for granted that schizophrenia is a biological illness. There is little argument that this disorder has a strong genetic predisposition, even if we do not know its precise mechanism. Yet a younger generation of psychiatrists might be surprised to learn that the question of the etiology of schizophrenia was once a battleground on which the forces of environmentalism suffered a severe defeat.

Freud (1910/1957) had believed that there was no point in attempting to treat schizophrenic patients with psychoanalysis, since, like most clinicians trained in the 19th century, he assumed that psychosis was constitutional. However, a younger generation of psychodynamically oriented therapists attempted to apply Freud's ideas to the understanding and treatment of the patients they were seeing in mental hospitals. Around the turn of the 19th century, a group of psychiatrists in Zurich became sympathetic to Freud's ideas, with Bleuler (1911/1950) and Jung (1921) proposing that psychodynamics can shape schizophrenic symptoms.

The ideas of this "Zurich school" met with resistance in Munich, where Emil Kraepelin was professor of psychiatry. The phenomenological school associated with Kraepelin's ideas dominated psychiatric thought in Europe. Kraepelin (1919) commented as follows on the early psychoanalytic theories of schizophrenia:

Here we meet everywhere the characteristic fundamental feature of the Freudian method of investigation, the representation of arbitrary assumptions and conjectures as assumed facts, which are used without hesitation for the building up of always new castles in the air, ever towering higher, and the tendency to generalizations beyond measure from single observations. I must finally confess that with the best will I am not able to follow the trains of thought of this "metapsychiatry," which, like a complex, sucks up the sober method of clinical observation. As I am accustomed to walk on the sure foundation of direct experience, my Philistine conscience of natural science stumbles at every step on objections, considerations, and doubts, over which the lightly soaring power of imagination of Freud's disciples carries them without difficulty. (p. 250)

Psychoanalysis had originally been designed for the treatment of neuroses. However, when psychoanalysis came to America, its practitioners became interested in applying its principles to a broader spectrum of patients. Many analysts suggested that it could be used to treat patients who today would be described as being prepsychotic or as having severe personality disorders (L. Stone 1954). Moreover, some psychoanalysts began to propose that schizophrenia itself might be primarily due to psychological factors.

Psychoanalytic theories about the childhood origins of schizophrenia were based not on studies of children but rather on historical reconstructions drawn from the therapy of adult patients. The purported early conflicts responsible for psychosis were therefore inferred but never observed.

We should realize that in the 1950s, psychiatry was very far from reaching our current standards for "evidence-based medicine." At that time, there were few systematic etiological studies of any mental disorder, and guidelines for clinical practice were based almost entirely on single case reports. In this climate, therapists could describe a few patients they had treated who had reported negative childhood experiences and then go on to theorize that these patients' illnesses developed because of those events. Many such papers were published in the best journals, and their authors could reasonably expect to impress their colleagues with their conclusions.

A common thread in many versions of psychodynamic theory is that the more severe the psychopathology, the earlier must be the stage of development from which it originates. This view stands in contrast to the principle advanced in this book: that the most severe forms of psychopathology have the strongest genetic loading.

An idea common among psychoanalysts interested in schizophrenia was that psychotic cognition is only one example of what Freud (1900/1953) had called "primary process," a normal thought process seen in infants or dreaming adults. Applying the theory of the primacy of early experience, some theorists (M. Klein 1946; Winnicott 1958) hypothesized that patients develop a psychosis rather than a neurosis because the historical roots of their conflicts occur *earlier in childhood,* even during infancy. Supposedly, this relationship between severe psychopathology and early experiences was based on "infant observation" (M. Klein 1946). In fact, Klein's observations consisted of nothing but the interpretations of an observer with a strong preconceived theory (Grosskurth 1986).

Another influential psychodynamic hypothesis was that psychosis is an attempt to escape from intolerable conflicts into an alternate reality (Fromm-Reichmann 1950; Sullivan 1953). In a similar fashion, theorists influenced by theories of family dynamics saw the symptoms of schizophrenia as attempts to avoid pathological family interactions. The best known of these theories, the "double-bind" model (Bateson et al. 1956), proposed that faulty communication patterns in a family cause psychosis, because thought disorder is the only way the patient has of escaping an impossible situation. The double-bind model never had a strong empirical base and is now thoroughly discredited (Gottesman 1991). Yet the enormous influence it had 30 years ago demonstrates how strong environmentalist thinking was at that time.

The "schism and skew" model (Lidz and Fleck 1985) is a rather similar idea, hypothesizing that pathological family structures cause schizophrenia by interfering with identity formation. Another related hypothesis is the famous construct of the "schizophrenogenic mother" (Arieti 1974; Fromm-Reichmann 1954). In this model, maternal psychopathology impinges on the child, so that overprotective and unempathic rearing practices eventually lead to psychosis.

Few of these ideas were ever subjected to stringent empirical tests. What research shows is that the only consistent feature of schizophrenic families is that they are more dysfunctional than normal families (Gottesman 1991). Even this observation could be accounted for by a shared biological vulnerability between parents and children or by the disruptive effects on family life of having a child with a psychotic illness. In summary, all attempts to identify any family pattern specific to schizophrenia have failed. No empirical findings have emerged in the last 25 years to challenge this verdict.

Today there is a wide consensus within psychiatry that schizophrenia has a strong genetic etiology. As pointed out by Kuhn (1970), paradigm shifts in science have their greatest influence on the younger generation. The old guard tend to stick to their earlier beliefs, and bad theories only die when their authors die. A good example is the idea that schizophrenia originates in family pathology. Long after this theory moved out of the scientific mainstream, its advocates continued to publish rear-guard critiques of the methods used to demonstrate biological factors in the illness (Lidz and Blatt 1983). Yet, as we will see later in this chapter, the evidence that schizophrenia is a genetically based illness has never stopped accumulating, leaving family theories of its etiology as historical footnotes.

■ Schizophrenia and Psychotherapy

Two historical factors were responsible for the upsurge of psychodynamic theories about schizophrenia. First, since psychodynamic ideas were already central to psychiatry, analysts were looking for new worlds to conquer. Second, the prognosis for the functional psychoses was much worse 40 years ago than it is today. To combat the hopeless fate of the chronic mental patient, almost *anything* was worth trying. Thus, psychotic patients were, at the same time, being treated with "heroic" methods of organic treatment, including frontal lobotomy (Valenstein 1986) or massive doses of electroconvulsive therapy (Collins 1988).

Forty years ago, when there was no consensus among psychiatrists about the need for clinical trials, one could report success in treating schizophrenic patients with psychotherapy without having to submit one's claims to serious empirical tests. The danger of practicing medicine without an evidence base is demonstrated by the work of John Rosen. "Direct analysis" (Rosen 1953) was a radical and rather "wild" form of psychoanalysis in which schizophrenic patients were confronted with immediate and "deep" interpretations about their supposed incestuous and aggressive wishes. Rosen created a fair amount of excitement in his time by claiming that his approach achieved dramatic cures of psychotic illness. Later, a careful follow-up of Rosen's patients (Bookhamer et al. 1966) demonstrated that these effects were nonspecific and transient, and that all of his patients had relapsed within a short time.

A good example of the climate of opinion about schizophrenia during the 1950s is the case of Joanne Greenberg. This patient was treated by the neo-Freudian analyst Frieda Fromm-Reichmann. Greenberg's own fictionalized account of her illness (Green 1964) became a best-seller and was later made into a successful film. The story, describing how a humanistic and compassionate therapist rescues a young girl from the prison of psychosis, had an understandably great appeal to the public.

As an adolescent, Greenberg developed an intense fantasy, bordering on a delusion, that she was living on another planet. Her condition led to her hospitalization at Chestnut Lodge, a private psychiatric hospital near Washington, DC. After a course of intensive psychotherapy, Greenberg recovered from her illness and became a highly successful writer. She continues to function on a high level in all aspects of her life (McGlashan 1989).

However, the Greenberg case is an example of the danger of generalizing single case reports of therapeutic success to larger clinical populations. McGlashan (1986), who followed up all of the patients admitted to Chestnut Lodge during the 1940s and 1950s, found that the schizophrenic patients did very poorly as a group. Even though the schizophrenia patients admitted to this hospital were a highly socioeconomically favored subsample, there was no indication that this population responded in any way to intensive psychotherapy.

Psychotherapy could be useful at a later point to help patients to recover from their illness. However, even this conjecture has never been proven in clinical trials. Rather, only the most practically oriented approaches, such as the teaching of social skills ("sociotherapy"), have been shown to reduce relapse rates (Hogarty et al. 1991, 1997).

Whatever effect psychotherapy has on the schizophrenic patient probably depends on "nonspecific" factors. In general, the effectiveness of any form of psychotherapy tends to be more associated with a good relationship with the therapist than with specific interventions (Garfield 1994; Strupp and Hadley 1979). A large-scale Boston study of the psychotherapy of schizophrenia (Stanton et al. 1984) was designed to compare psychodynamic therapy carried out over several years with long-term supportive therapy. The researchers found no difference whatsoever in outcome between the groups.

In the end, it was the success of pharmacological treatment and the failure of psychotherapy that turned the tide against environmentalist theories of schizophrenia. In one of the most influential studies (May 1970), when newly admitted patients were randomly assigned to drug treatment, psychotherapy, or a combination, only neuroleptic therapy led to adequate symptom control.

Finally, in evaluating any reported successes with psychotherapy in schizophrenia, one must be sure that patients actually merit the diagnosis. As shown by the famous New York–London study (Cooper et al. 1972), schizophrenia was, until about 25 years ago, being over-diagnosed in America, whereas mood disorders were being seriously underdiagnosed. Moreover, patients who today would be categorized as having personality disorders were being called either "ambulatory schizophrenics" (Searles 1965) or "pseudo-neurotic schizophrenics" (Hoch et al. 1962).

In the case of Joanne Greenberg, the original diagnosis remains uncertain. Greenberg was a subject in McGlashan's (1986) follow-up study, in which the subjects were rediagnosed with DSM-III criteria, and had met the criteria for both the schizotypal and borderline categories of personality disorder. Ironically, Greenberg may never have had schizophrenia.

In the light of our present knowledge, many of these past controversies seem quaint or archaic. Yet we must attempt to learn from the mistakes of the past and consider why these theories were so influential in their time in spite of the lack of any evidence to support them. Psychiatry is more committed to a scientific approach today. However, we should be humble enough to realize that our present theories may look equally out of date in another 50 years!

For the general public, the image of the schizophrenic patient as a misunderstood outsider and the idea that the illness can be blamed on bad parenting retain a wide appeal (Wessley 1997). Fortunately, hardly any contemporary psychiatrists share this perspective. Yet, as we will see later in this book, the same issues that made schizophrenia a battleground arise today in relation to other mental disorders. The ground may have shifted, but the idea that psychopathology is rooted in child-hood experience lives on.

Schizophrenia: The Evidence

We now have enough data to make quantitative estimates of the strength of the predisposition to schizophrenia. In summarizing our present state of knowledge, we will draw on two relatively recent comprehensive re-views of the literature (Black and Andreasen 1994; Gottesman 1991).

Behavioral genetic methods have been the key method for measuring the biological factors in schizophrenia. The concordance in monozygot-ic (MZ) twins ranges around 40%–50%, but is only about 10%–15% in dizygotic (DZ) twins. The heritability of the disorder is even greater when one takes into account that the first-degree relatives of probands often have disorders such as schizotypal personality that are really subclinical forms of schizophrenia (Kendler and Gruenberg 1984; Torgersen et al. 1993).

Adoption studies conducted in Scandinavia (Kety et al. 1975) have shown that if an adopted child has a schizophrenic biological parent, his or her risk for the disorder increases. The most recent adoption studies, conducted in Finland (Tienari et al. 1994; Wahlberg et al. 1997) and in Denmark (Kety et al. 1996), have found a similar degree of heritability. Again, schizophrenia has an even stronger genetic loading when we consider its "spectrum" as including individuals whose sub-clinical traits are markers for a predisposition to illness.

Studies of high-risk children also support the conclusion that schizo-phrenia involves a strong genetic predisposition. Cohorts of offspring of schizophrenic mothers have been followed for about 25 years and have been shown to be at much higher risk for both schizophrenia and schizophrenic spectrum disorders (Erlenmeyer-Kirling et al. 1995; Marcus et al. 1993; Mednick et al. 1988). Moreover, these individuals, even during childhood, show "soft neurological signs" similar to those seen in adult schizophrenic patients (Mednick 1987).

Thus far, research has failed to identify any specific biological marker associated with a diathesis to schizophrenia. The most consistent asso-ciation, to be discussed later in this chapter, involves abnormal eye movements.

Thus, in spite of massive research efforts, the precise biological nature of the genetic predisposition to schizophrenia remains unknown. The heritability data is most consistent with a polygenic mechanism of inheritance (Gottesman 1991). Recent research has suggested there may be specific loci of vulnerability on chromosomes 6 and 22 (Cardno and McGuffin 1996), but these findings have not been confirmed in all studies, and there may be different loci in different families (Maziade et al. 1997a). There may also be a different pattern of inheritance in early-onset versus late-onset cases (Maziade et al. 1997b). At this point, no specific gene loci are clearly associated with schizophrenia (Levinson et al. 1998).

The problem for researchers is that, contrary to the case for illnesses such as Huntington's disease, they cannot link their investigations of schizophrenia to an identifiable lesion (Kennedy 1996). We remain unsure about whether schizophrenia is one disease or many and about whether it can be separated from other psychoses. There is, in fact, evidence suggesting that the same genes can increase vulnerability for both schizophrenia and bipolar mood disorder (Crow 1995; Maziade et al. 1995). Moreover, it is more difficult to locate regulatory genes that influence complex events, such as neural connections during development, than to locate those that code for enzymes (Cloninger 1994).

Schizophrenia is somewhat more common and more severe in men than in women. In accord with a principle presented in Chapter 2, it is therefore not surprising to find that the illness is more familial in females (M. V. Seeman 1996). Genetic predispositions also vary with severity. The milder forms of schizophrenia, and the schizophrenic spectrum disorders, could derive from a less severe genetic loading. Finally, an early onset of schizophrenic illness is usually associated with a higher genetic loading (Gottesman 1991).

We do not know the mechanisms by which genetic variations affect brain function in schizophrenia. Genes operate on both neurophysiological and neurochemical levels. Unfortunately, our understanding of these processes, even in normal individuals, is still in its infancy.

The most influential current theory of the brain abnormalities in schizophrenia concerns abnormalities in dopaminergic transmission (Gottesman 1991). This theory helps to explain why pharmacological agents, including both the classical neuroleptics and clozapine, control schizophrenic symptoms by blocking different types of dopamine receptors (P. Seeman et al. 1987). Yet we do not really know whether receptor abnormalities cause schizophrenia or are the result of schizophrenia.

Neuropsychological abnormalities are found with some consistency in schizophrenic patients. A number of observations, including abnormal eye tracking and an aberrant P300 response on electroencephalography, suggest that schizophrenic individuals have particular difficulty integrating complex stimuli (Bilder 1996). Decreases in frontal lobe activation have been visualized in schizophrenic patients with positron-emission tomography (Andreasen 1984). Abnormalities in smooth-pursuit eye tracking (Holzman 1996; Litman et al. 1997) constitute a neuropsychological marker of particular significance, since such abnormalities are also found in the nonaffected relatives of schizophrenic patients. The same abnormalities also appear in related spectrum disorders such as schizotypal personality (Siever et al. 1990; Thaker et al. 1996).

Deficit symptoms in schizophrenia may derive from different mechanisms than do positive symptoms. The negative symptoms of the disease might be better markers of a genetic predisposition, and such symptoms are frequently accompanied by ventricular enlargement (Gottesman 1991). However, patients with deficit symptoms do not necessarily have a stronger family history of the disease (Tsuang et al. 1991).

Genetic factors may influence neural development, most particularly the migration of neurons during fetal life (Gold and Weinberger 1995; Weinberger 1987). It is possible that negative symptoms, particularly those associated with some degree of brain damage, reflect the effects of the environmental factors in schizophrenia, such as viral infections during fetal or perinatal life. Brain damage may also be responsible for the cognitive deficits in schizophrenia, which appear well before the onset of the disease. In an interesting example of a gene–environment interaction, estrogens have protective effects against the development of these symptoms, which helps to account for the fact that schizophrenia is less virulent in women (Tsuang et al. 1991).

One of the most influential current theories is that structural abnormalities in the brain precede the development of schizophrenic symptoms (Murray 1994). These changes would be associated with cognitive abnormalities that are probably developmental, deriving from connections between the frontal, temporal, and limbic areas (Gold and Weinberger 1995). Many of these connections develop during fetal life. Thus, any pathological influence that interferes with this process would increase the risk for schizophrenic illness. Crow (1995) suggests that lateralization makes the brain particularly susceptible to such insults.

Perhaps the most important unanswered question about schizophrenia concerns the precise nature of the environmental factors in its etiology. Heritability studies show that half of MZ twins are discordant for schizophrenia. This finding often reflects differences in the severity of the disorder, since unaffected twins are more likely to have schizotypal personality or other traits in the "schizophrenic spectrum" (Rosenthal 1971). When the full spectrum of these disorders is taken into account, clearer patterns of heritability are found (Kendler et al. 1993d). Thus, in a classical and still-fascinating study of identical quadruplets with schizophrenia (Rosenthal 1968), the severity of illness ranged from a single episode of positive symptoms to a chronic course accompanied by negative symptoms.

Some theorists (Strauss 1992; Zubin et al. 1992) have argued that psychological environmental factors also affect the severity of schizophrenic illness. However, the evidence suggests that disease severity depends either on the weight of genetic loading or on the presence of neurodevelopmental anomalies. Thus, the environmental factors in the etiology of schizophrenia are largely biological. Viral infection during pregnancy (Mednick et al. 1988), perinatal anoxia (Torrey et al. 1994), and Rh incompatibility (Mednick et al. 1988) all increase the risk for the disorder. The predisposition to schizophrenia is activated by a variety of factors that lead to brain injury (Wyatt 1991). Although genetic predisposition may increase sensitivity to these risk factors, it is brain injury that acts as the trigger, unleashing a process that uncovers the illness.

There is no evidence that problems in family life or in child development have any specific relationship to schizophrenia (Gottesman 1991). Family dynamics can, however, affect the *course* of the illness. The presence of "expressed emotion"—affectively charged criticism from relatives—influences the rate of relapse in schizophrenia (Falloon et al. 1984).

Social factors also play a minor role in the etiology of schizophrenia. This is shown by the nearly constant prevalence rate of the disorder around the globe (Jablensky et al. 1992; World Health Organization

1979). However, the *outcome* of schizophrenia shows important socio-cultural variability (Black and Andreasen 1994). The disease leads to much more severe dysfunction in the more economically developed countries. Although schizophrenia is found at about the same prevalences all over the world (Gottesman 1991), it is less chronic and more episodic in the less economically developed countries (Leff et al. 1992). The most likely explanation is that the stronger family and community supports in such societies act as protective factors. Even within North America, the Vermont Longitudinal Study (Harding et al. 1987) found many cases in which patients living in rural areas remained functional for surprisingly long periods. Schizophrenic individuals, or those with schizophrenic spectrum disorders, are therefore more likely to reproduce in traditional societies. On the other hand, in modern societies, where schizophrenia leads to more severe dysfunction, the fertility of affected individuals is low (Gottesman 1991). Meehl (1990) has hypothesized that for every case of overt schizophrenia, there could be many others in which "schizotaxic" or schizotypal traits are present without causing psychosis. In traditional societies, where marriages are arranged by families and where the social structure provides secure employment, such individuals may be fully functional. Yet in modern societies, people are expected to find their own mates and their own jobs. Those who are unable to meet these demands due to a genetic predisposition to schizophrenia are more likely to develop overt illness.

Summary

Few psychiatric disorders provide a better example of the predisposition–stress model than schizophrenia. Research continues, and we can expect to know much more about this illness within the next few decades. The following conclusions are in accord with our present knowledge:

1. Schizophrenia does not develop without a specific genetic predisposition.
2. This predisposition may express itself as full-blown illness or as disorders in the "schizophrenic spectrum."
3. The predisposition is more likely to result in illness in the presence of stressors that lead to brain injury.

9

Mood Disorders

The Boundaries of Depressive Illness

There is no clear cutoff point on the continuum between normal sadness and incapacitating depression. The inner experience of depression is familiar to many, and mild symptoms reflecting lowered mood are universal. Depressive affect is probably a biologically patterned response to loss, with the adaptive function of evoking help from other people (Bowlby 1980). Severe stressors can produce depression in virtually anyone.

In those who are unusually predisposed to depression, symptoms may appear with only mild environmental provocation. However, if a predisposition to depression is a widely distributed trait, then environmental factors should strongly affect the prevalence of depressive illness.

Mood disorders take many different forms; thus, to understand individual predispositions, we need an adequate classification. The boundaries of mood disorders have long been a source of confusion in psychiatry (Lehmann 1985). The most important unanswered question is whether depression is *one* disease, with various levels of severity, or *many* diseases, each with a different set of causes (Kendler and Gardner 1998). Thus, we do not know whether unipolar and bipolar depressions are different illnesses or represent different forms of the same illness.

We also do not know whether melancholic and nonmelancholic—or psychotic and nonpsychotic—depressions are more severe aspects of the same illness. Moreover, depression overlaps with a number of other psychiatric diagnoses with which it tends to be comorbid. Genetic epidemiological studies (Kendler et al. 1995a) suggest that neither the genetic nor the environmental factors in depression are specific, but rather that both overlap with risk factors for anxiety disorders, eating disorders, substance use disorders, and personality disorders.

Over the last 150 years, mood disorders have been classified in many different ways (Berrios 1992). In the last few decades, they have been dichotomized in various ways, none of which are very consistent with each other: endogenous versus reactive, psychotic versus neurotic, unipolar versus bipolar, major versus minor, and primary versus secondary. DSM-IV (American Psychiatric Association 1994) avoids some of these controversies by classifying disorders by means of their phenomenology. Ignoring the question of etiology, the system divides the group into unipolar and bipolar disorders and then distinguishes between melancholic and nonmelancholic depression.

By far the most commonly diagnosed mood disorder is major depression (L. N. Robins and Regier 1991). To make this diagnosis, we require, in addition to a depressed mood, the presence of five out of nine specific criteria associated with depression, and these symptoms must have been present for at least 2 weeks. This DSM definition can probably be recited from memory by many psychiatrists. It has the advantage of being reasonably precise and practically useful. The problem is that clinicians have come to *reify* this construct of major depressive disorder. The diagnosis of major depression is a *useful* way of describing psychopathology, but this does not make the construct "real"—nor can it, until we come to understand better the etiology and pathophysiology of mood disorders. (We will return to this problem in Chapter 16.)

The limitations of the construct of major depression are shown by the fact that a large number of permutations of symptoms can yield the same diagnosis. There are nine criteria, and although the patient must have either depressed mood or a loss of interest and pleasure, it is sufficient to have five of the others. This means that there can be more than 100 ways of meeting these diagnostic criteria. We should not think of depression as a unitary disorder.

Clinicians may also assume that making a diagnosis of major depressive disorder is a reasonable basis for a decision to prescribe antidepressants. In fact, DSM was never intended to be a treatment guide, nor is the claim made that diagnoses can guide the choice of therapy. The most useful guidelines for treatment involve subcategorizing major depressive disorder into melancholic and psychotic subtypes. These "five digit" diagnoses pick up the severity dimension that research shows is crucial for treatment selection. Melancholic depression usually responds to antidepressants, while psychotic depression often requires neuroleptics (Jefferson and Greist 1994). Many clinicians prefer to use dimensional scales, such as the Hamilton Depression Index (Hamilton 1960), to assess depression, so as to have a continuous measure of severity.

Depression, like schizophrenia, is a *spectrum* disorder. This means that the predisposition to become depressed varies in intensity and that its expression depends on environmental factors. The predisposition can express itself on a spectrum ranging from severe mental disorders to characterological variations (Akiskal et al. 1980). At one end of the spectrum lies incapacitating illness, such as recurrent unipolar depression with melancholic and/or psychotic features, while at the other end is depressive personality, characterized only by a pessimistic outlook on life (Phillips et al. 1990). The majority of cases take an intermediate form.

The depressive spectrum is not smooth and continuous. We can still find peaks and valleys, representing qualitatively different forms of illness. There could be multiple thresholds for depression, each reflecting different forms of illness. Thus, melancholic and nonmelancholic depressions could each have a different weighting of risk factors, with predispositions playing a stronger role in the melancholic type and stressors playing a greater role in the nonmelancholic type.

A good deal of empirical evidence supports this hypothesis. The more severe the depression, the more likely it is to involve a positive family history (Nurnberger and Gershon 1992). Twin studies show higher concordances in patients with recurrent unipolar illness than in unipolar patients who have had fewer than three episodes (60% vs. 30%). Twin studies also show that severe depressions are more heritable (Lyons et al. 1998). Recent negative life events are more likely to be found in patients without melancholic symptoms (G. W. Brown et al. 1994; E. Frank et al. 1994).

■ Genetic Predispositions to Depression

Twin studies have consistently shown that mood disorders are heritable (Gershon 1990; Nurnberger and Gershon 1992). The heritability is higher for bipolar illness. In the largest-scale study conducted to date (Bertelsen et al. 1977), the monozygotic (MZ) concordance for bipolar illness was nearly 80% (much higher than in schizophrenia), while the concordance in dizygotic (DZ) twins was only 25%. On the other hand, the MZ concordance for recurrent unipolar illness in the same sample was only about 50% (close to the rate in schizophrenia) with a DZ concordance of 19%. The researchers also noted that in MZ pairs concordant for mood disorders, the twins can have either bipolar *or* unipolar illness. This seems to suggest a common predisposition underlying both disorders, but this conclusion may apply *only* to the recurrent and severe forms of unipolar depression.

Although twin studies support the heritability of unipolar depression, adoption studies have yielded less conclusive results. In the best-designed study conducted to date, Mendelewicz and Rainer (1977) found that the morbid risk for affective illness was no greater in adopted-away children of parents with mood disorders than it was in adopted children whose biological parents did not have mood disorders. In this study, heritability became statistically significant only when depressive spectrum disorders ("minor depression" and dysthymia) were included.

The precise mechanism for genetic predispositions to mood disorders is unknown. For example, earlier proposals that bipolar disorder is transmitted through a gene on specific chromosomes (e.g., X or 11) failed to find sufficient support (Gershon 1990). Recent evidence from linkage studies for a susceptibility gene on chromosome 18 (Berretini et al. 1997) requires confirmation.

The relationship of the genetic factors in depression to age at onset is unclear. In line with the theory presented in Chapter 2, an early onset of depression would be expected to be a marker for stronger genetic factors in the etiology of the illness. Some studies (reviewed in Gershon 1990) have supported this principle, while others (Kendler et al. 1992d) have not. In the case of depression, environmental factors also influence age at onset, with some forms of depression with onset in old age being more heritable than depression occurring earlier in life (Gatz et al. 1992).

Research on depression occurring in children and adolescents has also yielded contradictory findings. Thapar and McGuffin's (1994) twin study found a stronger genetic component in depression that began in adolescence. Yet, in another study of adolescent twins (Rende et al. 1993), environmental factors better accounted for the more severe levels of depression. In the study of Thapar and McGuffin (1994), depression beginning before adolescence was associated with a strong environmental component (derived from the "shared" risk factors), pointing to family dysfunction as an etiological factor.

Neither is the course of depression consistently related to its heritability. Recurrent unipolar disorder is no more strongly inherited than single episodes, and rapid cycling bipolar disorder is no more strongly inherited than non–rapid-cycling types (Gershon 1990).

The most likely explanation of these confusing findings lies in the heterogeneity of depression. The presence of genetic effects in some cases could be blurred by the predominance of environmental effects in others.

With regard to the heritability of depressive illness, the most consistent finding in the literature is that severe depression is more heritable than mild depression. Although twin studies (Kendler 1997a) suggest that melancholia may be only a more severe form of depression, the presence of neurovegetative symptoms is linked with increased heritability (Kendler et al. 1992d). Genetic factors are also stronger in depressions that lead to hospitalization (McGuffin et al. 1991, 1996). Thus, different mechanisms may be involved in depressive illness at differing levels of severity (Kendler et al. 1996).

Dysthymia is a mood disorder in which symptoms are chronic but milder than those in depression. Dysthymia responds to antidepressant therapy rather less predictably than does major depressive disorder (Kocsis et al. 1991). Akiskal et al. (1980) have suggested that the category of dysthymia is heterogeneous and includes both milder cases of depression and cases in which chronic lowering of mood is associated with a personality disorder.

This raises a question: when does chronic depression distort personality, and when does personality pathology cause chronic depression? The comorbidity of any form of depression with a personality disorder predicts chronicity (Alnaes and Torgersen 1997). It is also interesting to note that dysthymia is comorbid with personality disorders in more than 60% of cases, three to four times greater than the comorbidity of major depression with personality disorders (Pepper et al. 1995). Moreover, when depression and dysthymia have an early onset, they are even more strongly comorbid with Axis II disorders, particularly those in Cluster B (Fava et al. 1996; Riso et al. 1996).

In the mildest forms of depression, predispositions may be expressed not as overt illness but as personality traits. These traits can still be precursors of major depression. A large body of research (Coyne and Whiffen 1995) points to two personality traits that increase the likelihood that environmental stressors will lead to depressive illness. The first of these, called "sociotropic" or "dependent" traits, characterize individuals who are unusually sensitive to loss or abandonment. The second, called "autonomous" or "self-critical" traits, describe individuals who are unusually sensitive to failure to achieve their goals. Like other traits, these personality characteristics are themselves genetically influenced, as shown by their correlations with broader personality dimensions such as neuroticism (Coyne and Whiffen 1995).

In summary, depression is heterogeneous. Some cases of depression show a strong genetic component, while others demonstrate stronger environmental influence. In the future, we may have clear-cut biological markers to identify the predisposition to mood disorders. These might help us develop better ways of subtyping mood disorders, thereby increasing our ability to disentangle the effects of nature and nurture.

The Role of Stressors in Mood Disorders

Predisposition–stress theory helps us to avoid the fruitless debates so common in the past as to whether depressions are "endogenous" or "reactive." They can be, and usually are, both.

There need not be *specific* stressors associated with the onset of mood disorders. Stressful events can also be biological, as in cases where "secondary" depressions arise after a medical illness (F. K. Goodwin and Jamison 1990). More commonly, stressors are psychological. Research demonstrates increases in the number of major life events occurring prior to the onset of affective episodes (Paykel and Cooper 1992). However, it is not clear whether these events are a cause of illness or a consequence of its early stages.

One of the psychological stressors most frequently thought to lead to depression is interpersonal loss (Bowlby 1980). Psychiatrists have long assumed that pathological grief is an important cause of clinical depression. However, clinicians may sometimes be mistaken in attributing cause and effect to this sequence of events. For every case in which depression follows bereavement, there are many others in which it does not. There is actually only weak empirical evidence that recent losses increase the risk for depressive episodes (Paykel and Cooper 1992).

Another widely held but questionable belief is that loss early in life represents a risk factor for depression later in life. Although this has been a controversial area of research, several careful reviews of the literature (Paykel and Cooper 1992; Tennant 1988) have concluded that there is no consistent evidence demonstrating that childhood losses actually increase the risk for adult depression.

Some years ago, G. W. Brown and Harris (1978), in a widely quoted study, reported that the early loss of a mother was an important risk factor for depression in women. However, subsequent studies have either failed to replicate this association or have shown it to be less important than other risks (Parker 1992). For example, in a large-scale twin study, Kendler et al. (1991) found that loss of a parent prior to age 17 explained only 2% of the variance in the development of major depression.

Another commonly held idea is that emotional neglect of children by their parents increases the likelihood that children will become depressed later in life. Parker (1983) has found that depressed patients consistently report that their parents were both neglectful and overcontrolling, a pattern Parker terms "affectionless control." However, these findings are based on the retrospective perceptions of patients who are currently depressed and therefore more likely to see the past in a negative light.

For parental neglect and overcontrol to be considered as etiological factors in depression, children suffering parental neglect and overprotection would have to be prospectively followed into adulthood to see if they developed mood disorders. Some prospective studies (reviewed in Rutter 1985) suggest that such parental styles may indeed be associated with increased depression in offspring. Rutter concluded that of all possible childhood adversities, a consistent lack of affection in childhood is the only consistent risk factor for nonmelancholic adult depression.

But in general, the importance of recent and remote life events in the etiology of mood disorders has been somewhat exaggerated. As discussed in Chapter 3, children usually remain resilient in the face of a wide range of adversities. As we will go on to discuss in Chapter 11, resilience is also the rule for adults dealing with serious trauma. These findings support the general principle that negative events have different effects on predisposed individuals.

The prevalence of mood disorders varies a great deal with gender. Although bipolar illness affects men and women equally, unipolar depression is about twice as common in women (Weissman et al. 1988). Is this a genetic difference, an environmental difference, or both?

One possibility is that gender differences could be an artifact, since women are more likely to verbalize their feelings, while men are more likely to use alcohol to avoid experiencing painful emotions. In a study of the Amish (Egeland and Hostetter 1976), in whom substance abuse is quite rare, depression was found to be equally prevalent in men and women. Nevertheless, Weissman and Klerman (1985) concluded that since sex differences in depression have been observed in many countries around the world, they are probably real.

We know of no sex-linked genetic factors determining the threshold for depressive illness. Nevertheless, in view of the well-known effects of hormones on mood (Halbreich et al. 1992), it seems likely that hormonal fluctuations are one of the factors that make women more vulnerable to depression.

In addition, differential prevalence may be rooted to some degree in psychosocial factors that differentially affect males and females. Women in early adulthood have a high prevalence of many forms of mental disorder (L. N. Robins and Regier 1991). One of the most important correlates of depression in women is an unhappy marriage (Weissman et al. 1988). These effects may be less strong if women have other sources of self-esteem. Thus, epidemiological research (Srole 1980) suggests that as women are entering the work force, their mental health is getting better, not worse.

One of the most striking research findings concerning depression is the increase in its prevalence over recent decades. This *cohort effect* has been well established in American samples (Klerman and Weissman 1989; L. N. Robins and Regier 1991) and has also been observed in other countries (Cross-National Collaborative Group 1992). Interestingly, the findings also apply to some extent to bipolar illness, which has also been showing an increasingly early age of onset.

When a mental disorder becomes more common over a short period of time, the explanation cannot depend on changes in predispositions, but rather must reflect an increase in stressors. Moreover, rapid cohort changes in stressors over a single generation are unlikely to be purely psychological, but are much more likely to be social.

What changes in the social environment could lower thresholds for depression? If depression were a biologically programmed system to maintain attachment bonds (Bowlby 1969), then any social change that interfered with attachment would increase its prevalence. The most likely candidates would therefore be increased rates of family break-down, and/or a breakdown in community structures outside the family, leading to compromised social networks. The effects of social stressors would also be mediated by gene–environment interactions. Thus, subpopulations who are already prone to mood disorders may account for cohort increases in their prevalence (Gershon and Nurnberger 1995).

Another line of evidence for the importance of social factors in depression is the cross-national differences in its prevalence (Weissman et al. 1996). In a population-based survey conducted in 10 countries, the lifetime prevalence of major depression ranged from 1.5% (in Taiwan) to 19% (in Lebanon). There were also differences among the most modernized societies, with a rate of 5% in America, as compared with rates ranging between 9% and 12% in Germany, Canada, Italy, and New Zealand. The prevalence of bipolar illness was much more stable than that of unipolar illness, but depression had similar symptoms, age at onset, and gender distribution in all of the countries studied. Only environmental factors can account for these striking findings.

■ Gene–Environment Interactions in Mood Disorders

Without a diathesis, negative life experiences and difficult interpersonal relationships do not necessarily cause depressive illness. Yet without stressors, the predisposition to depression may never become activated.

In a large-scale community study of adult female twins, Kendler et al. (1993e) examined genetic and environmental factors in individuals with unipolar depression. The best-fitting model, which predicted about half of the variance in liability to major depression, described interactions between a heritable component and a strong influence from psychosocial stressors.

Gene–environment interactions make any model of the causes of depression more complex. Stressful life events are only weak predictors of mood disorders and may even reflect indirect genetic influences, since those who are predisposed to depression are more likely to experience negative events (see Chapter 3). For example, those who become easily depressed by virtue of their diatheses are also more likely to have difficulties with their interpersonal relationships. Psychological research suggests that pessimists are often more realistic about life (Lewinsohn et al. 1980). However, pessimism can also bring on negative life events through a mechanism of "self-fulfilling prophecy."

Recent research (Shea et al. 1992) has shown that depression is a more chronic illness than was previously believed. One likely explanation involves a "kindling" theory of depression (Post 1992). In this model, environmental events change the biological mechanisms that lead to mood disorders. Each time a person becomes depressed, it lowers the threshold for predispositions to express themselves on future occasions, so that less severe stressors are subsequently required to uncover them. Therefore, stressors might play a more important role in the *early* stages of mood disorders, with negative events increasing sensitivity to further episodes.

Unipolar depression is a high-prevalence disorder (L. N. Robins and Regier 1991). As with most highly common disorders, it is also heterogeneous. Melancholic depression can take severe, life-threatening forms, while mild depression can be thought of as "the common cold of psychiatry." If the predisposition to depression is widely distributed in the population, this would help explain why environmental changes, such as the social factors implicated in cohort effects, can cause dramatic changes in the frequency of depressive illness.

Both schizophrenia and bipolar illness involve a "spectrum." Relatives of affected probands often have milder forms of these disorders or only trait variations that need not lead to significant dysfunction. These observations help to explain why the traits underlying these disorders remain in the gene pool. There could even be a role for balanced polymorphism in some major mental illnesses. There is evidence, for example, that the first-degree relatives of patients with mood disorders are unusually energetic or creative (Andreasen 1987).

In depression, having a diathesis is probably a necessary but not a sufficient condition for developing overt illness. The life events preceding a depressive episode tend to be those that would be stressful for anyone, and these stressors lead to only mild or temporary impairments in most people (Paykel and Cooper 1992). On the other hand, in those with a depressive diathesis, the same events lead to major psychopathology (Kendler et al. 1995b). Without stressful events, a diathesis may never become manifest.

Individuals prone to depression may have specific personality traits, termed "neuroticism"—that is, high levels of pessimism and worry that actually make negative life events more likely (Kendler et al. 1993c). Since mood and anxiety disorders are highly comorbid (Maser and Cloninger 1990), it is not surprising that traits of neuroticism are also associated with anxiety disorders.

Unlike schizophrenia, unipolar depression shows large cohort differences in prevalence within the same society (Klerman and Weissman 1989). This observation points to the importance of social factors in its etiology. Further support for this conclusion comes from studies of the genetic epidemiology of depression (Kendler et al. 1992d), which show that the environmental components in these disorders are "unshared" and therefore related to the larger social environment. Social stressors can make individuals with a diathesis to depression cross the threshold into clinical symptoms (G. W. Brown and Harris 1989).

▓ Summary

The following conclusions seem consistent with the present evidence about mood disorders:

1. Among the mood disorders, bipolar disorder is associated with the strongest genetic predisposition.
2. Severe depressions (i.e., those with melancholia and/or psychosis) will not occur in the absence of genetic predispositions.
3. Milder cases meeting the criteria for major depressive disorder are associated with predispositions of lesser intensity.

4. The milder the depression, the more important the role of environmental factors in its etiology.
5. Shared environmental factors deriving from the family environment can be important risk factors in certain subgroups, particularly children.
6. There is only a tenuous relationship between life events, such as early or recent losses, and the development of a depressive illness.
7. There is no simple causal relationship between stress and depression.

10

Anxiety Disorders and Other "Neuroses"

The experience of anxiety is universal. Like depression, anxiety is a biologically programmed response to environmental stress, functioning to mobilize the organism to deal with danger (Bowlby 1969). Yet some individuals have lower thresholds than others for developing anxious feelings. We need to understand the origins of mental disorders in which anxiety loses its link with precipitating circumstances. Moreover, we need to explain how anxiety takes so many different forms: the terror of a panic attack, the constant worry of generalized anxiety disorder, the specific fear of phobia, or the irrational thoughts of obsessive-compulsive disorder.

In this chapter, we will also examine, albeit rather more briefly, other symptomatic disorders that present somatically rather than as overt anxiety. In previous editions of DSM, these diagnoses were classified with the anxiety disorders, among the "neuroses." Although the tenth edition of the *International Classification of Diseases* (ICD-10) (World Health Organization 1992) continues to maintain this grouping, in DSM-III (American Psychiatric Association 1987) these categories were detached from their neighbors because of differences in phenomenology. Yet all of these disorders may share common predispositions, with social factors determining how distress is expressed (Kirmayer et al. 1994a).

■ Predispositions to Anxiety Disorders

Both panic disorder and generalized anxiety disorder (GAD) have a significant heritable component. The most important evidence for this conclusion comes from twin studies. Torgersen (1983) was the first to use DSM criteria in examining twins with anxiety disorders. Panic symptoms showed the greatest heritability, with a concordance of 31% in monozygotes and only 6% in dizygotes. These findings were later confirmed in another study from the same research group, this time using a much larger sample (Skre et al. 1993). Similar findings also emerged from a large population-based sample of American women (Kendler et al. 1993b). In general, the heritability of panic disorder is at about the same level as that of unipolar depression.

Kendler et al. (1992b) also examined the heritability of GAD. The precise level of heritability depends on whether one takes into account the comorbidity of this diagnosis. The concordances for "pure" GAD, i.e., without panic or depression, were 35% in monozygotic twins and 12% in dizygotic twins.

The mechanisms of inheritance for anxiety disorders are unknown. Segregation analyses of families of patients with panic disorder do not show any conclusive pattern, and attempts to find genetic linkages for anxiety disorders have thus far been unsuccessful (Knowles and Weissman 1995).

As discussed in Chapter 9 in relation to mood disorders, one of the problems in studying predispositions is our uncertainty about the validity of the boundaries between our diagnostic entities. It is not clear whether there are any absolute differences between the anxiety disorders themselves or between anxiety disorders and mood disorders.

For this reason, it is difficult to determine whether the boundaries between predispositions correspond to the boundaries described in our classification system.

Given the striking phenomenological differences between panic disorder and generalized anxiety disorder, one might conclude that panic symptoms derive from a different type of biological vulnerability. Thus, panic disorder occurs in discrete episodes, whereas GAD is continuous. Panic patients are characterized by anticipatory anxiety and by the complication of agoraphobia. Differential responses to pharmacological treatment also support the DSM distinction between these two conditions (D. F. Klein et al. 1985).

Yet behavioral genetic research does not really support a sharp boundary between panic disorder and GAD. Kendler et al. (1987) reported a large overlap in genetic predispositions between the two disorders. Thus, we still do not know whether these diagnoses are two different illnesses or different forms of the same illness.

In many ways, generalized anxiety functions more like a trait than a disorder. GAD might therefore have the same relation to acute anxiety as dysthymia has to depression. Like dysthymia, which is in most cases associated with an Axis II diagnosis (Pepper et al. 1995), GAD has also been shown to be highly comorbid with personality disorders (Blashfield et al. 1994).

Another question concerns whether panic disorder and major depression have different phenomenologies but derive from a common predisposition. The two disorders certainly have a substantial comorbidity (Goldberg and Huxley 1992; Maser and Cloninger 1990; Weissman et al. 1993). Drawing on evidence from family studies, Weissman (1993) concluded that panic disorder and major depression are independently and specifically transmitted. On the other hand, as with panic disorder and GAD, behavioral genetic findings do not support a sharp separation between anxiety disorders and mood disorder. Thus, in a large sample of female twins, Kendler et al. (1987) found that predispositions to both panic disorder and GAD show a strong overlap with predispositions to depression. Similar conclusions emerged from a recent study based on a Swedish twin registry (Roy et al. 1995). Kendler et al. (1987) have proposed that anxiety and depression may derive from the same genes but may present with different symptoms because they are associated with different environmental stressors.

Until we understand the biological underpinnings of anxiety and depression, we cannot definitively describe their relationship. It would be of great theoretical interest, however, if it turns out that a common trait predisposition can be shaped into different, albeit overlapping, symptomatic patterns. (We will be examining other possible examples of this principle in future chapters.)

One might expect the predispositions to anxiety disorders to be apparent before the development of overt illness. As is usually the case for depression, anxiety disorders tend to appear for the first time in adulthood. Yet, at least in some individuals, predispositions consisting of anxious traits can be observed early in life—even during infancy.

Social anxiety can be identified in young children by the presence of an unusually strong fear of strangers or of new situations. Kagan (1994) has termed this temperamental variation "behavioral inhibition." The presence of these traits in childhood probably increases the risk for anxiety disorders in adulthood (Rosenbaum et al. 1993), although long-term follow-up of children with these characteristics is needed to confirm this hypothesis. It is also likely that behaviorally inhibited children are at greater risk for anxious-cluster personality disorders in adulthood (see Chapter 15).

Stressors in Anxiety Disorders

As with mood disorders, stressors may not have a specific relationship to anxiety disorders. Underlying traits can be activated by a variety of stressors. Recent negative life events often precede the onset of symptoms, acting as triggers for the onset of overt disorders.

In a large clinical sample of patients with panic disorder or agoraphobia, Lteif and Mavissakalian (1995) found a significant association between recent stressful life events and the onset of symptoms. Similar findings, applying to both panic disorder and generalized anxiety disorder, emerged from a large-scale community study in Canada (Newman and Bland 1994).

The direction of causation between life events and anxiety is not clear. For example, in the Lteif and Mavissakalian study, negative events were strongly related to an underlying personality dimension: neuroticism, a trait already known to have a large heritable component. As discussed in Chapter 3, personality traits influence the quality of life events, and frequent negative experiences in life can reflect as much about predispositions as they do about stressors. Another possibility is that anxiety disorders, like mood disorders, might demonstrate "kindling." Thus, Farvelli and Pallanti (1989) reported that recent negative life events are most common before the *first* episode of panic disorder, and lower levels of stress might be required to reactivate panic symptoms once they have already occurred.

In parallel with the discussion of the psychological factors in depression in Chapter 9, the direction of the relationship between anxiety disorders and childhood experiences is unclear. Attachment theory (Bowlby 1973) predicts that individuals prone to anxiety should have suffered more experiences of threatened or real separation and loss early in life. However, this "intergenerational transmission" of attachment patterns might have other explanations. "Anxious attachment" also depends on personality traits that are common to parents and children. Until we can identify the biological markers for anxious traits, it will be difficult to disentangle the effects of nature and nurture.

Retrospective research seems to suggest that adults with anxiety disorders have had serious difficulties in early family life. For example, patients with anxiety disorders are more likely to remember their parents as both neglectful and overprotective (Parker 1983). However, interpreting these findings is difficult. First, retrospective patient reports may reflect the tendency of individuals with serious present difficulties to describe the past as problematic. Second, problems in parental behaviors are not specific to anxiety disorders, given that very similar reports come from patients with mood disorders, personality disorders, and many other psychiatric diagnoses. After reviewing this literature, Parker (1992) concluded that there is no *proven* relationship between events in childhood and anxiety symptoms in adulthood.

We can best interpret these data as supporting the hypothesis that predispositions determine whether patients are prone to panic disorder or GAD, whereas stressors determine when the threshold of liability is crossed. Shear et al. (1993) have proposed a psychodynamic theory of panic disorder in which an anxious temperament leads to a vulnerability to panic disorder, which is then amplified by problems with parents—in particular, excessive criticism that interferes with the development of self-esteem. In vulnerable individuals, panic symptoms would ultimately be precipitated by life stressors, especially those producing frustration and resentment. Although this theory contains a number of speculative elements, it takes into account interactions between predisposition and stress.

Obsessive-Compulsive Disorder

Obsessive-compulsive disorder (OCD) has had an interesting history. The radical changes in how clinicians have viewed this condition over time resemble the story of schizophrenia presented in Chapter 8.

Fifty years ago, obsessions and compulsions were conceptualized within a psychodynamic framework as defenses against intrapsychic conflicts. Freud (1909a/1955) famously described the successful analysis of a patient with OCD, influencing future generations to be optimistic about the use of psychotherapy for these symptoms. However, the illness of this patient, referred to as "the rat man" because of his obsession with rats, was not a very typical example of OCD. For one thing, his symptoms were of recent onset, unlike most patients, who develop OCD in childhood or adolescence (Rapaport 1989). We will also never know whether the rat man's symptoms would have relapsed with time, because he was killed early in the First World War.

OCD can be a chronic and disabling disease. Severe cases of OCD are usually unresponsive to psychotherapy and may improve only with high doses of clomipramine or serotonin reuptake inhibitors (Rapaport 1989). These observations have led contemporary psychiatrists to think of OCD as a primarily biological illness.

Yet the genetic factors in OCD remain unknown. There have been no twin or adoption studies of this disorder, nor have family history studies identified any clear pattern of inheritance. Black et al. (1993) examined the relatives of OCD patients and found no higher frequency of OCD. Instead, and rather surprisingly, there was a greater prevalence of personality disorders.

However, several other lines of evidence (reviewed in Hollander et al. 1994) support the hypothesis of a genetic–biological component in OCD. These include abnormalities on neuropsychological testing, abnormal findings on neuroimaging, electroencephalographic changes, and associations between OCD-like symptoms and lesions of the basal ganglia. As Stanley and Wand (1995) have pointed out, OCD has a stable cross-cultural prevalence, which, as in the case of schizophrenia, supports the assumption that it involves a large biological component.

One of the complicating factors in OCD is that, like other anxiety disorders, it is probably etiologically heterogeneous. For example, recent evidence (Dar 1996) suggests that treatment is generally more effective in late-onset than in early-onset cases. This finding could suggest a relationship between an early onset of illness and a stronger biological predisposition (see Chapter 2). Moreover, as in the case of unipolar depression, severity of illness, ranging from severe and chronic to mildly episodic (Jenike 1995), might also reflect differences in genetic loading.

Much remains to be learned about OCD. We do not understand the genetic predisposition associated with this disorder. We also need to undertake systematic studies of the role of environmental factors in the development of obsessive and compulsive symptoms.

Phobias

Phobias are among the most prevalent of all psychiatric diagnoses (L. N. Robins and Regier 1991). However, most cases do not come to clinical attention. This is probably because phobic situations can often be readily avoided, so that the patient escapes significant dysfunction.

Freud (1909b/1955), describing the treatment of a 5-year-old boy, suggested that phobic symptoms could be symbols for internal conflicts. In contrast, Watson (1926/1970) saw phobias as conditioned responses that are determined by exposure to environmental stressors. However, neither psychoanalytic nor behavioral theory explains individual differences in the susceptibility to phobias.

Bowlby (1969) took a more biologically grounded view of this problem. Following Darwin, he noted that phobias are exaggerations of normal fears. Although some phobias are clearly irrational, what most children are afraid of would usually have constituted *real* threats in the environment of evolutionary adaptiveness (i.e., the environment of Paleolithic man). Thus, fears of heights, of animals, or of strangers are all potentially adaptive responses. Bowlby thought that phobias present clinically only when there is concurrent anxiety about separation from a caretaker who is needed to protect the child from these dangers.

Attachment theory has, however, failed to account for two issues: 1) why are there individual differences between children in their susceptibility to specific fears? and 2) why are different children afraid of different things? Biological predispositions could provide the answer to these questions.

Thus far, only a few studies have examined the heritability of phobias. In a clinical sample of twins, Skre et al. (1993) found that simple phobias and social phobias were not heritable at all. Yet, in a much larger community sample of female twins, Kendler et al. (1992c) found the heritability of phobias to fall within about the same range as that of other anxiety disorders—i.e., 30%–40%. The explanation for this disparity could be that researchers usually find greater heritability in community samples, since there are always many more individuals who carry a predisposition than there are those who manifest clinical symptoms.

Kendler et al. (1992c) have reported different degrees of heritability for different subtypes of phobia. Genetic factors were most important for animal phobias, although fear of an animal usually requires some degree of traumatic exposure. On the other hand, in spite of the fact that agoraphobia is often a complication of panic disorder, genetic factors were somewhat less important in this type of phobia.

In summary, phobias have a moderately strong genetic component. Whether or not predispositions develop into overt symptoms usually depend on stressors, in some cases involving direct exposure to a fearful situation and in others depending on nonspecific stressful circumstances.

Other "Neuroses"

Somatization Disorder

Somatization disorder, a diagnostic construct characterized by chronic and multiple physical symptoms, has replaced the older term, "hysteria," traditionally used to describe such patients. (I will discuss below whether this change in terminology constitutes a real improvement.)

Some family history studies (Cloninger 1986) have suggested that somatization disorder aggregates in the female relatives of female probands, whose male relatives are more likely to develop antisocial personality disorder. This association remains controversial, although one adoption study (Bohman et al. 1984; Cloninger et al. 1984; Sigvardsson et al. 1984) supported an inherited tendency to somatization linked to both antisocial personality and alcoholism in men. There have been no twin studies of somatization disorder.

As Kendler et al. (1995a) concluded, the relationship between genetic factors and somatic symptoms is not very specific. As with anxiety disorders, similar traits seem to underlie many different types of psychopathology. Thus, the tendency to somatize can be seen in somatization, conversion, and hypochondriacal disorders. All of these symptoms are also related to personality dimensions, particularly to neuroticism, or "negative affectivity" (Kirmayer et al. 1994a). Both of these traits are known to be heritable. It should therefore not be surprising that somatization disorder is highly comorbid with personality disorders (J. Stern et al. 1993).

There are also important psychosocial determinants of somatization. Expressing distress somatically can be the result of a socialization process, so that children learn, through reinforcement and modeling, to use bodily rather than cognitive means to display their feelings (Kirmayer et al. 1994a).

Conversion Disorder

Like OCD, conversion disorder has a long and interesting history in 20th-century psychiatry. Freud (1909c/1953) described a famous case, "Dora," a young woman who developed physical symptoms as a result of being caught in the web of a dysfunctional family. The *Dora* case actually documented an unsuccessful course of treatment but was published to illustrate the purported psychodynamics behind conversion symptoms.

What psychoanalytic theory fails to explain is why some patients develop conversion symptoms while others, with similar difficulties, develop totally different neurotic symptoms. The traditional explanation assumes the presence of a specific conflict or developmental fixation. There is little evidence to support these hypotheses. No one has been able to show empirically that the psychological issues faced by patients with conversion disorders are in any way different from those faced by patients with other types of neurosis. Moreover, the personality characteristics that Freud believed to be associated with developmental "fixations" have not been shown to derive from experiences or problems at any particular stage of childhood (S. Fisher and Greenberg 1996).

There has been hardly any formal research on conversion disorder. We do not know whether there exists a specific predisposition to conversion symptoms or to somatization in general. As in anxiety disorders and depression, it possible that a general predisposition could be shaped into different symptoms in different social contexts (Shorter 1994).

To some extent, conversion can be learned behavior. Transcultural research sheds significant light on how symptoms are shaped by social factors. Conversion symptoms are much more prevalent in less economically developed countries and have been among the most common presentations in mental health and primary care clinics in India (Nandi et al. 1975). However, this situation is changing. A group of researchers examined symptomatic presentations in a clinic in a Bengali village, first in the 1960s (Nandi et al. 1975) and then in the 1980s (Nandi et al. (1992). They found that the prevalence of conversion symptoms declined markedly over this 20-year period. (Over the same period, suicide attempts increased dramatically, raising the question of whether the same pathology underlies both somatization and impulsive self-harm.) Similar findings, describing decreased rates of conversion disorders over time, have been reported in the United Kingdom (Leff 1988) and in Greece (Stefanis et al. 1976).

These data demonstrate how social change can shape vulnerabilities to psychopathology into different symptomatic presentations. As clinicians, we may sometimes forget that symptom clusters are not necessarily "real" entities. All diagnostic entities reflect some degree of social shaping, and environmental differences can elicit different symptoms from the same predisposition.

We might therefore reopen the case concerning the validity of the construct of "hysteria." At the end of his career, the great British psychiatrist Sir Aubrey Lewis remarked (A. Lewis 1975): "a tough old word like hysteria dies very hard. It tends to outlive its obituaries" (p. 12). Yet outside a few centers, one hardly ever hears this term used. Many feel that we are well rid of the term, given that the original construct (based on the Greek word for "womb") applied almost exclusively— and often inappropriately—to women.

Since DSM-III, psychiatry has divided hysteria into conversion, dissociation, and somatization (Kihlstrom 1994). The decision to do so was based on the principle that unless there is clear evidence that smaller entities fall within larger clusters, we should generally favor splitting over lumping of diagnoses. Merskey (1995) has argued for the retention of the older construct. Hysteria describes a pattern of symptoms that can be malleable and mercurial. The construct also describes patients who are highly suggestible and whose symptomatology responds to whatever is current in the social environment. Thus, patients attending medical clinics will show somatic symptoms, while patients influenced by what is current in the media may have a wide range of presentations, possibly including parasuicide or dissociation.

In discarding hysteria, something has been lost. Even feminist writers (e.g., Showalter 1996) have revived the term to describe psychological or somatic syndromes. But if we bring back the construct, we will clearly need to assign it a different name!

Summary

All of the disorders discussed in this chapter (panic disorder, generalized anxiety disorder, obsessive-compulsive disorder, phobia, somatization disorder, and conversion disorder) fit the predisposition–stress model. The major problem for further research in this area concerns the limits of the present diagnostic classification. When we know more about the biological mechanisms behind these disorders, we will probably find ourselves understanding them in a different way.

11

Posttraumatic Stress Disorder

The Construct of Posttraumatic Stress Disorder

The fact that traumatic experiences can have long-term effects has been known throughout human history. These phenomena can even be found in such classical sources as Homer's *Odyssey*.

However, the description of a specific medical syndrome associated with trauma did not appear until the 19th century, largely as a result of observations on the effects of combat during the American Civil War (Trimble 1985). Since then, posttraumatic symptoms have been described by clinicians after each of the conflicts that have marked our own century. In the First World War, the effects of combat exposure were called "shell shock." In the Second World War, a similar syndrome was called "combat fatigue." The experiences of psychiatrists working with Vietnam veterans led to the present construct of posttraumatic stress disorder (Wolf and Mosnaim 1990). In recent years, there has been a strong revival of interest in all sorts of trauma as causes of psychopathology (McFarlane 1996).

Symptoms similar to those seen in war veterans have also been documented in many other groups: survivors of the Holocaust (Sigal and Weinfeld 1989), noncombatants during wartime (Yehuda et al. 1996), and children exposed to trauma (Terr 1988). The most characteristic symptoms that can follow trauma have become the defining features of a new category first listed in DSM-III (American Psychiatric Association 1980).

Posttraumatic stress disorder (PTSD) is primarily defined by recurrent intrusive recollections and a sensitivity to environmental events that resemble the original event. In DSM-IV (American Psychiatric Association 1994), posttraumatic reactions are subclassified by their time course: symptoms lasting less than 1 month are termed "acute stress reaction," symptoms lasting up to 3 months are termed *acute PTSD,* and symptoms lasting more than 3 months are termed *chronic PTSD.*

A large amount of research has been published in the last few decades about PTSD. However, much of this research suffers from two serious problems: retrospective methodology and comorbidity.

Retrospective Methodology

In most studies of PTSD, exposure to trauma has been measured retrospectively, not prospectively. As we will see later in the chapter, this is a critical problem with all trauma research. As discussed in Chapter 9, retrospective perceptions of life experience are usually influenced by present levels of symptomatology. Thus, when we ask veterans who are currently symptomatic about their war experiences, they may be more likely to describe them as traumatic.

In a recent study, Southwick et al. (1997) followed Gulf War veterans prospectively and found that those who continued to have symptoms tended to remember their war experiences as more traumatic over time. These fascinating findings raised such serious questions that the published report of the study was accompanied by an editorial titled "What is PTSD?" (Hales and Zatzick 1997).

Comorbidity

As Young (1995) has noted, most war veteran psychiatric patients meet criteria for many other psychiatric disorders, particularly depression and substance abuse. Southwick et al. (1993) have reported that personality disorders are unusually prevalent in this population. In addition, we cannot ignore the role that compensation plays in the continuation of posttraumatic symptoms in veterans. Yet despite these complexities, some clinicians attribute the morbidity of these patients almost entirely to their history of trauma.

A Predisposition–Stress Model of PTSD

Posttraumatic stress disorder is one of the few categories in the DSM classification to have a putative etiological agent built into its definition. Yet, as we will see, there is no simple causal relationship between trauma and PTSD.

There are also several problems with the PTSD construct itself. First, how do we define *trauma*? This term has been overused to the point that almost any negative life event can be called "traumatic." We would be better advised to call events traumatic only when they consistently lead to negative effects. Yet, as we will see, even the most disastrous life events do not inevitably lead to pathological sequelae.

Second, how do we define *stress*? This rather vague term has been used to describe a wide variety of environmental challenges (Kirmayer 1996). Yet, as discussed in Chapter 3, the stressfulness of events strongly depends on the personality of the exposed person. Therefore, calling an event "stressful" need not imply that the event necessarily involved circumstances totally beyond the individual's control.

As recently pointed out by Yehuda and McFarlane (1995), PTSD was introduced into the classification of mental disorders to validate the experiences of trauma survivors. However, psychopathological sequelae are not always attributable to the nature of the traumatic event. It is not true that *all* individuals exposed to trauma develop posttraumatic symptoms. In fact, the evidence shows that traumatic events do *not* by themselves consistently produce PTSD, even when such events are severe (Breslau et al. 1991).

As reviewed by Yehuda and McFarlane (1995), what the data show is that the *short-term* effects of trauma are mediated largely by the nature of the traumatic event. In contrast, *long-term* effects (i.e., PTSD) are mediated by factors specific to the individual. Thus, the category with the highest prevalence among exposed populations would be acute stress disorder. Acute PTSD should be much less common, and chronic PTSD even less so.

Combat exposure is a good example of these basic principles. In the short run, participating in combat usually produces some psychological symptoms. However, most war veterans, even those who have been in life-threatening battles, never develop PTSD. In fact, of those exposed to combat, only 25% ever develop the full clinical picture described in DSM (Laufer et al. 1984).

What determines who develops PTSD and who does not? To some extent, the *severity* of trauma is a factor. However, the association between combat exposure and later symptomatology is not very strong (Fontana and Rosenheck 1994; Helzer et al. 1979). Lee et al. (1995), in a 50-year follow-up of World War II veterans, found that although severity of combat exposure predicted acute PTSD, long-term symptoms were strongly related to premorbid psychopathology.

As discussed in Chapter 3, personality affects the *frequency* of negative life events, thereby influencing both exposure and susceptibility to stressors. Thus, factors intrinsic to the individual could be among the most important determinants of whether trauma leads to PTSD. Individual differences even influence whether traumatic experiences happen at all. Breslau et al. (1991) found that traumatic events are more likely to befall individuals with certain personality traits, particularly high neuroticism and high extraversion. Soldiers with antisocial traits are more likely to be exposed to danger, from which they emerge either as casualties or as heroes (Yochelson and Samenow 1976).

A second factor determining vulnerability to trauma concerns overall predispositions to psychopathology. One of the strongest predictors of PTSD in war veterans is a personal history (King et al. 1992; Solomon et al. 1988) or a family history (Kettner 1972) of psychiatric illness.

Behavioral genetic research has provided support for the hypothesis that predispositions influence whether combat veterans develop PTSD. In a very large sample of twins who served in the Vietnam War, True et al. (1993) reported differences in concordance between monozygotic and dizygotic twins for each of the specific symptoms of PTSD. In the same sample (Lyons et al. 1993), even the degree of combat exposure itself showed strong heritability, most probably because of the strong genetic component in risk-taking behavior.

If *all* of the symptoms of posttraumatic stress disorder are heritable, PTSD cannot be a simple consequence of exposure to stress.

There are two overall conclusions we can draw about combat exposure:

1. Severity of exposure is only moderately associated with PTSD risk.
2. PTSD depends on interactions between predispositions and stressors.

The occurrence of PTSD following disasters has allowed researchers to apply prospective methodologies in which the severity of exposure to the traumatic event can be measured at baseline instead of being assessed retrospectively years later. In his classic study of Australian fire fighters, McFarlane (1990, 1993) found that the longer symptoms remained, the less they were accounted for by exposure to trauma and the more they were accounted for by predispositions. Vulnerability to PTSD depended on personality traits of neuroticism or conflict avoidance as well as on either a family history or a personal history of psychiatric illness.

A retrospective community study by L. N. Robins et al. (1981) showed that individuals with *chronic* PTSD associated with a variety of traumatic events had most of the same predisposing factors described by McFarlane. Atkeson et al. (1982) have reported similar findings following exposure to violent crimes. Finally, in a community study of individuals exposed to a wide variety of stressors, Skre et al. (1993) found that PTSD was highly heritable.

In summary, the symptoms of PTSD usually result from the triggering of pathology to which the individual is already predisposed or an exacerbation of symptoms that had previously been present. Research indicates that although *acute* PTSD can often be accounted for by exposure to trauma, *chronic* PTSD cannot. Chronicity derives from predisposing factors, and resilience factors can protect exposed individuals against chronicity (Flach 1990). The data clearly support a predisposition–stress model of PTSD.

Histories of Childhood Trauma in Psychiatric Patients

When trauma occurs at a defined moment in time, the course of posttraumatic symptoms can then be followed prospectively. If, on the other hand, traumatic events have occurred at some point in the past, we can only assess them retrospectively. Given the effects of all possible intervening events, it becomes very difficult to attribute psychopathology to temporally distant stressors. This problem raises serious doubts about claims—based entirely on retrospective studies—that childhood trauma consistently causes PTSD or that traumatic events in childhood lead to predictable long-term psychopathological sequelae.

A large number of studies applying retrospective designs have claimed to document associations between childhood trauma and adult psychopathology. For example, personality disorder patients (see Chapter 15), dissociative disorder patients (Spiegel and Cardena 1991), and somatization disorder patients (Kirmayer et al. 1994a) all report high rates of childhood sexual and physical abuse. Such reports might be interpreted as demonstrating that childhood trauma is indeed an important risk factor for the development of adult psychopathology. However, it is equally possible that these associations have no etiological significance whatsoever.

Community surveys of the long-term sequelae of childhood trauma help to put these issues into perspective. The great majority of survivors of child abuse (about 80%) have *no* measurable psychopathology (Browne and Finkelhor 1986; Malinovsky-Rummell and Hansen 1993). Thus, many more nonpatients than patients have trauma histories.

A recent large-scale community study in New Zealand (Fergusson et al. 1996a, 1996b) reported somewhat higher rates of childhood sexual abuse than most North American studies, yet serious sequelae remained rare. Taking into account methodological problems such as recall bias and latent variables, the authors concluded: "the weight of the evidence points to the conclusion that childhood sexual abuse may play a significant, but not overwhelmingly strong, role in determining individual vulnerability to psychiatric disorder" (Fergusson et al. 1996b, p. 1372).

On the whole, research on trauma in children resembles that reviewed earlier on PTSD in adults. Exposure to trauma is a necessary but not a sufficient condition for the development of symptoms, with resilience remaining the rule.

These findings are important, and we need to explain them. We must keep in mind that any associations between abuse history and adult pathology are correlational and could be explained by other coexisting psychosocial or biological risks. However, the sequelae of abuse depend very much on severity of exposure. Trauma is not one thing, but many things. Therefore, in order to understand the impact of any experience, we must consider its *parameters*.

Severity of exposure is an important predictor of the long-term effects of many adverse experiences during childhood (Rutter 1987a). Associations between childhood sexual abuse or physical abuse and psychopathological symptoms in adult life are much stronger when the parameters of the abuse experience are taken into account (Browne and Finkelhor 1986; Malinovsky-Rummell and Hansen 1993).

By far the most powerful predictor of sequelae in childhood sexual abuse is father-daughter incest, which leads to negative consequences in about half of cases (Russell 1986). Negative consequences are also significantly more likely if the perpetrator of the sexual abuse is a member of the child's family, if the abuse is frequent and occurs over a long period, if force is applied, and if penetration takes place (Browne and Finkelhor 1986). However, with the important exception of father-daughter incest, even when these severity parameters are taken into account, most studies indicate that the majority of children exposed to sexual abuse will *not* develop significant psychopathology.

To review the argument presented in Chapter 3, single traumatic experiences in childhood do not usually lead to mental disorders, whereas multiple negative events lead to cumulative effects that significantly increase the risk for psychopathology. Any one negative event in childhood interacts with many other life experiences. To the extent that other experiences are positive, the child will be more likely to show resilience to trauma. To the extent that other experiences are also negative, the effects of the event will be amplified. Thus, if we fail to note that traumatic events co-occur with many other risk factors, associations between single events and psychopathological sequelae can give us the mistaken impression that isolated incidents have enormous consequences.

This principle has been clearly demonstrated in community surveys of child abuse. Many of the symptoms associated with childhood sexual abuse can be accounted for by the effects of coexisting risks, such as overall family dysfunction and the absence of maternal affection (Fromuth 1986; Nash et al. 1993; Rind et al. 1998). Clinical samples yield parallel findings: in L. N. Robins' (1966) classic prospective study examining which children with conduct disorder go on to develop antisocial personality disorder, physical abuse alone had no predictive value unless that abuse was perpetrated by an antisocial parent living in the home.

The long-term effects of childhood trauma therefore support the principle that when children suffer adversities, resilience is the rule. As discussed in Chapter 3, positive experiences can act as protective factors when they buffer negative experiences. In particular, the presence of positive attachments *outside* the family affords a high level of protection against risk factors *inside* the family (Kaufman et al. 1979). Research on the long-term outcome of childhood sexual abuse has shown that its sequelae depend strongly on the quality of other relationships and experiences in the child's life (Romans et al. 1995).

In summary, the long-term effects of trauma during childhood are not simply a function of exposure. Coexisting risk factors are crucial to outcome. Moreover, predispositions explain why the same risk factors can produce psychopathology in one individual but not another.

The Accuracy of Memories for Traumatic Events

Psychopathological theories based on trauma models explain a variety of adult symptoms as long-term reactions to childhood events. These models are based on the primacy of early experience (see Chapter 3) and do not take account of predispositions. Theories that attribute a wide range of adult symptoms to childhood trauma also contradict the evidence that most people exposed to such trauma develop few long-term symptoms, and that most people with serious psychological symptoms have not been exposed to trauma.

Since so many of their patients lack a history of childhood trauma, many therapists committed to these theories have come to believe that even in the absence of reports of traumatic events, such events *must* have occurred. This belief has led some therapists to search for "repressed memories" (Merskey 1995). As a result, a great controversy has arisen. Serious questions exist regarding whether, and the extent to which, patients' memories of trauma in childhood are credible.

The question of the accuracy of long-term memory must influence our interpretation of any purported associations between negative childhood experiences and adult psychopathology. The problem arises quite often in clinical practice. Given the vagaries of human memory, the historical data we obtain from our patients, which depends on accurate memory for events that occurred many years in the past, must always be regarded with caution.

Research shows that most memories of past events are not reports but reconstructions (Bartlett 1932/1995; Loftus 1979; Paris 1996b). Spence (1992) has termed the distinction between how we remember things and what "really" happened "narrative versus historical truth." Clinicians deal *only* with narrative truth. The way we construct our experience depends on individual differences in personality traits and cognitive styles.

This principle applies no matter how much emotion accompanies a reported memory. It has been shown that memories of past events that are *known* to be false can nonetheless be reported with great conviction. False memories also tend be full of telling details that can convince the inexperienced observer that they must be accurate. In experiments in which memories were implanted through suggestion (Loftus 1979) or through hypnosis (Laurence and Perry 1983), the researchers noted that there was no way, other than by independent corroboration, to distinguish false from true memories. The power of suggestion is much greater than most clinicians realize. Suggestion also explains how false memories of childhood events can be stimulated by the expectations of therapists who search for traumatic events (Loftus 1993).

The problem of false memories is one good reason that reports of child abuse in adults should ideally be corroborated by other observers (Brewin 1996; Esman 1994). Surprisingly, very few studies of trauma in psychiatric patients have attempted to establish such corroborative evidence. Some researchers have used sibling reports as validators, although in one study in which siblings were asked to confirm patients' reports of childhood events, there was only fair agreement regarding events such as deaths and separations and very little agreement as to perceptions of family atmosphere (L. N. Robins et al. 1985).

The way we remember things, as well as the way we explain what has happened to us, is very much a function of our personality. It is not surprising, therefore, that when behavioral geneticists examine standard self-report instruments used to elicit childhood experience in twins, many of which purport to be measures of the environment, they find that a substantial heritable component affects scores on all of these scales (Plomin and Bergeman 1991).

Some aspects of parents' child-rearing practices may be more affected by the child's personality than others. Thus, studies in which twins reported on how their parents raised them (Kendler 1996; Rowe 1981) found a large heritable component in how adults remembered parental affection but not in how they remembered parental control. The most likely explanation for these findings is that positive temperamental characteristics in *children* elicit more affection from parents, whereas the methods by which parents control their children reflect the personality traits of *parents*.

Clinicians need to understand the problems with the accuracy of recollections before coming to firm conclusions about the validity of historical material presented in psychotherapy. The development of false memories in psychotherapy is a very real possibility. It is unlikely that patients intentionally fabricate experiences of abuse, and patients with false memories are not actually *inventing* traumatic histories. Rather, recollections of their experiences are shaped by suggestions coming from many sources (Loftus 1993). These include books, media, and previous therapists, all of which can and do influence patients to believe in the reality of repressed memories.

To place this problem in a scientific context, let us now review the research literature on the overall accuracy of human memory. A large number of studies (reviewed in R. A. Baker 1990; Bowers and Hilgard 1988; Orne et al. 1988; Pettinati 1988; Schacter 1996) yield conclusions that will be surprising to many clinicians:

1. Normal memories are not necessarily accurate.
2. There is no intrinsic way to distinguish true from false memories.

There are several different types of memory. Remembering data such as a telephone number, or noting the route to a specific location, involves different mechanisms than recalling events. We must therefore develop classifications of memory that take into account the difference between remembering facts and remembering events. Researchers have used different terms to emphasize this separation: *semantic* versus *episodic* memory, *explicit* versus *implicit* memory (Schacter 1996). The important point is that factual memories are more accurate than event memories. All event memories involve serious distortions.

These observations make more sense when we consider the *functions* of memory. The brain is continuously bombarded with environmental input, so that what is recorded requires screening. Memory formation must focus on the encoding of only the most salient aspects of events. Moreover, what is encoded is then processed, so that the ultimate record of events reflects the influence of cognitive schemata. As a result, memories always contain some degree of *confabulation*. In effect, what we remember is the outcome of an interaction between events and cognition. This principle applies at the time of registration, at the time of memory recall, and at all intervening times.

All memories involve some degree of imaginative reconstruction. This applies to how we remember every type of experience. One might think that emotion-laden events would be remembered more vividly. Some theorists (e.g., van der Kolk 1994) have proposed that traumatic memories are laid down in a special way in the brain that makes them more accurate. However, studies of "flashbulb memories," either for important events in one's own life or for socially meaningful events such as the assassination of a famous person, demonstrate that such memories are consistently distorted by individual preconceptions (R. A. Baker 1990; Ofshe and Watters 1994).

Thus, contrary to the belief of some clinicians, memory does *not* function like a tape recorder. What is laid down is an overall impression that is generally, not factually, precise. The details of events are not recorded, but instead tend to be added after the fact. The unreliability of memory has been demonstrated in many studies examining the accuracy of eyewitness testimony (Christianson 1992; Loftus 1979).

If memories are not laid down in detail in the first place, verifying them does not involve "accessing records" in the mind. In many cases, there is no way to determine precisely what happened in any event. This conclusion should come as no surprise to historians!

Some therapists are under the impression that hypnosis makes memories more accurate. In fact, the reverse is true. Memories obtained under hypnosis are much more likely to be false. Empirical studies have shown that the highly detailed memories of past events that can be elicited or implanted under hypnosis, which seem at first to be convincing evidence for the "tape recorder" theory of memory formation, are based largely on fantasies and can often be understood as a response to the expectations of the hypnotic situation (Laurence and Perry 1983; Orne et al. 1988; Spanos 1982). It is for this reason that courts in most jurisdictions do not admit as evidence memories that have emerged only under hypnosis (Gutheil 1993).

Childhood Trauma and Repressed Memories

The theory behind the use of hypnosis in "recovering" memories is that consistent trauma leads to the *repression* of memory for these events.

Terr (1991) hypothesized that when children are traumatized, particularly by caretakers on whom they are dependent, they need to use defense mechanisms to cope with these experiences. By repressing any memories of the trauma, they might, in the short run, cope better.

These ideas can be traced back to Freud's (1896/1962) original theory of repressed memory. His view was that when traumatic events cross a stimulus barrier, they cause painful anxiety, and that repression represents an attempt to defend against this anxiety. The hypothesis that repressed memories from childhood are a cause of adult psychopathology was originally proposed by Breuer and Freud (1893–1895/ 1955) to account for conversion symptoms; in their "Studies on Hysteria," they stated that "hysterics suffer mainly from reminiscences."

In recent years these issues have again become a source of controversy. Psychoanalysts such as Masson (1984) and Miller (1984) have criticized Freud for attributing psychopathology to oedipal fantasies rather than to real experiences, and for suppressing the facts about child abuse. It has also become apparent through community research that childhood sexual abuse is much more common than had previously been thought (Finkelhor et al. 1990; Russell 1986). Clinicians have taken an interest in patients who have experienced either incest (Herman 1981) or other forms of childhood sexual abuse (Herman 1992).

The long-term effects of child abuse on adults has entered the consciousness of the general public through best-selling books (e.g., Bass and Davis 1988). Unfortunately, these popular tracts have offered a great deal of misleading information about the effects of abuse and repressed memories (Loftus 1993). They have also probably influenced many patients, particularly those who are highly suggestible, to believe that they were abused as children even when they cannot remember such events.

There is surprisingly little experimental evidence for the repression of memory (Bower 1990; Holmes 1990; Pope and Hudson 1995). Since repression is an elusive phenomenon, it may be difficult to demonstrate its existence through experiments. It is possible that an experimental situation is not a good model for the traumatic conditions under which memories might become repressed. For ethical reasons, there has been little formal research as to whether traumatic events actually cause the repression of memory. Thus, in spite of the lack of evidence in its favor, repression is a hypothesis that cannot easily be refuted.

A recent report by Meyer-Williams (1994) seems to provide the first scientific evidence that traumatic memories can actually be repressed. In this study, individuals known to have been abused as children were followed up as adults and interviewed to determine the extent to which they were aware of those past events. The main finding was that 38% of women with documented sexual abuse during childhood failed to mention having experienced these events.

However, questions arise about the interpretation of these findings (Pope and Hudson 1995). At first glance, the results are consistent with a theory of repression after trauma. Yet even when the subjects did not recall the specific episode that was reported to child protection authorities, most remembered *other* incidents of abuse. Only a few (12%) remembered no abuse at all, and among these, most incidents occurred before age 5, a time when few individuals have many reliable memories. Finally, in a parallel study, Femina et al. (1990) found that subjects who *seemed* to forget incidents of abuse during adolescence actually preferred not to discuss these events with researchers, although they could describe them when specifically asked.

The most parsimonious conclusion from the current research is that repression of traumatic events probably does occur but is quite exceptional.

In a famous first sentence of a highly influential book, Herman (1992, p. 1) claimed: "The ordinary response to atrocities is to banish them from consciousness." Statements of this kind are provocative but ignore decades of clinical experience and research showing that PTSD is usually associated with painful recollection of traumatic events. Forgetting is most certainly *not* the usual result of trauma.

Observations in adults consistently show that when individuals are followed for various periods of time after known traumatic events, they do *not* repress memories (Horowitz 1993). On the contrary, particularly if they develop PTSD, they tend to have continuous and intrusive thoughts about these events. What does frequently happen after trauma, however, is the conscious *suppression* of memories, a process that probably allows for more effective coping (Wyshak 1994).

Some theorists have asked whether the mechanisms of dealing with trauma are any different in children. Terr (1988) conducted a classic study showing that posttraumatic symptoms in children are phenomenologically similar to symptoms in adults. When children were followed after a traumatic experience (kidnapping on a school bus), they *tried* to suppress their memories but continued to be troubled by them, and they embroidered their memories of the event with many false details.

Ironically, it was also Terr (1991) who later proposed that *chronic* trauma, particularly abuse perpetrated by a caretaker, interferes with memory access. Terr suggested that such "Type II trauma," as she labeled it, might be identified by hallmarks such as denial, numbing, dissociation, and chronic anger. However, no prospective studies of chronically traumatized children have documented such a mechanism. Retrospective studies of trauma cannot be used to prove the existence of this phenomenon, since, as we have seen earlier, traumatic memories are often difficult to verify. Nor is there any evidence that the symptoms Terr describes as associated with Type II trauma can be used as validators, since they do not have a specific relationship to trauma. If anything, the evidence is more consistent with a contrary hypothesis: when traumatic memories *are* repressed, they are *most* likely to involve single incidents and *least* likely to arise under conditions of long-term abuse.

Is Dissociation a Marker for Trauma?

Spiegel (1990) has suggested that a failure to remember traumatic experiences could involve *dissociative* mechanisms. In this view, trauma can cause entire sectors of the mind to become blocked from consciousness.

Unfortunately, dissociation has proved even more difficult to measure than repression. Researchers have had to evaluate the construct indirectly, through symptoms that are assumed to reflect such a mechanism. Dissociative phenomena consist of disturbances of memory, excessive mental absorption, and depersonalization (Carlson 1994). These symptoms are known to be more common in individuals with documented exposure to acute traumatic events who have subsequently developed PTSD (Spiegel and Cardena 1991). Patients with dissociative disorders often describe histories of severe trauma during childhood (Spiegel and Cardena 1991).

There are three overall problems with these claims for an association between dissociation and trauma. The first concerns our definition of dissociation. Many studies have used measures, such as the Dissociative Experiences Scale (DES; Carlson 1994), that are not very specific to what has classically been described as dissociation and that are heavily weighted with questions that might be better thought of as measures of general psychopathology. For example, one of the symptoms most strongly associated with recent trauma is psychic numbing. However, it is not clear in what way this symptom is specifically "dissociative," since numbing is also associated with anxiety disorders (Merskey 1995).

A second problem with these claims concerns the validity of the "dissociative disorder" construct. This category reifies dissociative processes that are common to many forms of psychopathology (Kirmayer 1994a). It is not clear why the presence of dissociative symptoms should define a separate group of mental disorders. This provides an excellent example of the problem of separating psychiatric syndromes from disorders. Attempts to assess dissociative disorders more precisely founder on the essential problem of whether the construct itself is valid. For this reason, neither self-report instruments (e.g., the DES) nor semistructured interviews (e.g., the Structured Clinical Interview for DSM-IV Dissociative Disorders [Steinberg 1994]) used to make these diagnoses prove their validity (Paris 1996d; Piper 1997).

The third problem with the claims that dissociation and trauma are associated concerns the reports of childhood trauma from the patients studied by researchers investigating dissociation. But in every case, these reports are entirely retrospective, lacking any independent verification. Moreover, these reports of trauma often consist of highly questionable "recovered memories" that have been either elicited under hypnosis or strongly suggested by therapists treating these patients (Paris 1996d; Piper 1997). There have been no prospective studies in children that support the hypothesis that dissociative symptoms are rooted in traumatic experiences.

In addition, the associations between trauma and dissociation described in clinical populations might be accounted for by latent variables. For example, these links may be due to family dysfunction and not to child abuse (Mulder et al. 1998; Nash et al. 1993). Some researchers (e.g., van der Kolk et al. 1991) have found associations between trauma histories and dissociation or self-mutilation in patients with personality disorders. However, when our own group studied dissociation in a similar population (Zweig-Frank et al. 1994a, 1994b, 1994c, 1994d), scores on the DES were strongly associated with a diagnosis of borderline personality disorder but were not, independently of that association, related to histories of trauma.

As a result of these findings, our group hypothesized that dissociation in borderline personality disorder might depend more on heritable traits than on childhood experiences. To pursue this idea, we studied DES scores in a twin sample to determine whether they are heritable. The findings of this study were that both overall DES scores and DES subscale scores show highly significant levels of heritability (Jang et al. 1998). Butler et al. (1996) have suggested that the capacity to dissociate may also be linked with hypnotizability, a personality dimension that has long been known to be heritable.

The capacity to dissociate is therefore most likely a *trait* that can be amplified to pathological proportions by psychosocial stressors. In spite of the purported links between dissociation and trauma, these symptoms may not have any specific relationship to environmental experiences. As was originally hypothesized by Janet (1907), the development of dissociative symptoms requires both predisposition and stress.

Nor have researchers explained why trauma should cause dissociation in some patients and not others. For example, surprisingly few features of dissociation have been observed in survivors of the Holocaust, a group with well-documented severe psychic trauma (Yehuda et al. 1996).

Moreover, dissociative symptoms, like somatic symptoms, are strongly shaped by cultural factors. Transcultural studies suggest that in certain societies, dissociation is a culturally sanctioned way of expressing psychic distress (Kirmayer 1996).

It follows from this discussion that neither dissociation nor any other specific symptomatological pattern identified thus far can be used to confirm the validity of memories for childhood traumatic experiences.

Summary

Posttraumatic stress disorder, which at first glance appears to fit an environmental model of psychopathology, instead turns out to demonstrate the necessity for a predisposition–stress model.

However dramatic the symptoms in trauma victims, and however de-serving these patients are of our sympathy and concern, we need to ad-dress the role of underlying predispositions in PTSD. Genetic factors are crucial determinants of whether traumatic events will have long-term effects. The same principle applies to adult patients who report childhood trauma. Traumatic stressors do not usually produce lasting psychopathology on their own, but instead act to unleash preexisting vulnerabilities.

The clinical implications of this research are profound. Clinicians need to keep in mind that most people are resilient to trauma. They should therefore be cautious in explaining the causes of mental disor-ders through either recent or distant life events.

12

Substance Abuse

S ubstances are chemicals that alter mental activity. Only humans consistently use substances that were not available in the environment in which they evolved.

Predispositions and stress each play important roles in the etiology of substance abuse. Alcohol is by far the most commonly abused substance, and this form of substance abuse has been the subject of the largest quantity of research. Therefore, this chapter will focus on alcoholism research.

Predispositions to Substance Abuse

The essential elements of brain chemistry are similar in all vertebrates and evolved early in the history of the vertebrate phylum. As a result, substance abuse is one of the few mental disorders for which researchers can develop animal models (Lumeng et al. 1995). The pharmacological effects of substances largely depend on their ability to tap into existing neurochemical mechanisms. A striking example of this parallelism is provided by the exogenous opioids, which act on the same brain systems as endorphins (Snyder 1978).

Genetic differences in brain function lead to differences in individual responses to substances. Ultimately, predispositions to substance abuse reflect neurochemical and neurophysiological variability. One of the main lines of evidence supporting this view is that individuals who later become dependent on substances find them pleasurable the first time they are exposed to them, whereas those who are less likely to become subsequent abusers find the same substances initially unpleasant (D. W. Goodwin 1985). The "level of reaction" (Schuckit and Smith 1996) to alcohol—that is, how much one has to drink to become intoxicated—has also been shown to be a predictor of future abuse.

There are several possible ways to understand why individuals prefer one substance over another. In the first hypothesis, a "lock and key" relationship exists between differences in neurochemical configuration and preferences for a substance. Khantzian (1985) has hypothesized specific relationships between preferences for substances, personality traits, and neurochemical variability. Thus, individuals whose neuropsychological makeup leads them to require *increased* levels of stimulation may prefer activating substances such as cocaine, while those who need to *reduce* their stimulation levels may favor opioids. Khantzian's theory does not account for polysubstance abuse, which is associated with significant Axis II comorbidity (DeJong et al. 1993).

A second hypothesis suggests that a common predisposition operates in many types of substance abuse. This trait has been called "addictive personality" (D. W. Goodwin and Warnock 1991). According to this theory, individuals who are susceptible to substance abuse suffer from chronic dysphoria, which leads them to use drugs as a form of self-medication. In this view, addiction develops when hyperreactivity to stress is specifically buffered by the intake of a substance. As we will see, this hypothesis is supported by research studying the sons of male alcoholics, a group at very high risk for substance abuse (Pihl and Peterson 1990).

A third possibility is that substance abuse is linked to traits of impulsivity. In this view, the crucial factor in addiction is the inability to control intake. Impulsive traits could also help explain the high comorbidity between substance abuse and personality disorders (DeJong et al. 1993).

A fourth possibility is that the choice of a substance is largely determined not by specific predispositions but rather by sociocultural factors. As we will see in the next section, there is a good deal of evidence supporting this hypothesis.

Sociocultural Factors in Substance Use

Some form of substance use is seen in every society. However, sociocultural factors often determine the choice of substance and the extent to which it is abused.

Alcohol has been and continues to be the substance of choice in most cultures throughout human history. However, other substances have also presented serious problems (Westermeyer 1991). In the past, opioid dependence was highly endemic in China, and it remains a major source of addiction in North America and Europe. After a long period of declining use, cocaine has again become a serious clinical problem in Western countries.

Cultural norms encourage substance use by associating intake with reinforcing interpersonal activity. The primary example consists of the male-bonding rituals associated with drinking in many societies. Cultures can also discourage substance use, either by enforcing sanctions and prohibitions against abuse or by associating its use with activities in which the role of the substance is secondary, such as taking alcohol only with meals.

Alcoholism

Alcoholism is heterogeneous. Different forms of alcohol abuse are associated with different predispositions and are elicited by different stressors (Hesselbrock 1995). Moreover, when a disorder is extremely prevalent, it is more likely to derive from several different etiological pathways. In the case of alcoholism, epidemiological studies in North America have demonstrated a prevalence of 14% in males (L. N. Robins and Regier 1991).

Many years ago, Jellinek (1960) hypothesized that alcoholism takes several different forms, some having a later onset and being less familial and others having an earlier onset and being more familial. A contemporary version of this classification emerged from adoption studies of alcoholism conducted in Scandinavia (Bohman et al. 1987; Cloninger et al. 1981; Sigvardsson et al. 1996). The findings pointed to two independently heritable types of alcohol abuse. "Type 1 alcoholism" has a later onset, affects both sexes, and is determined by both genetic and environmental factors. "Type 2 alcoholism" has an early onset, affects only men, is associated with criminality, and is more strongly determined by genetic factors.

Predispositions

There are no clear cutoff points between increased consumption of alcohol, problem drinking, and clinically diagnosable alcoholism. Most likely, each of these levels of alcohol abuse is shaped by predispositions. Large-scale population-based twin studies, both in America (Kendler et al. 1992a, 1994) and in Australia (Heath et al. 1997), have demonstrated that problem drinking has a genetic component. Although the American findings were limited to women, the Australian sample had twins of both sexes. The results of that study showed that genetic factors account for approximately half of the variance in the average weekly consumption of alcohol and in histories of problem drinking. However, the findings of a Canadian twin study (Jang et al. 1995) suggested that severe alcoholism carries a higher genetic load.

Additional evidence for a biological predisposition to alcoholism comes from the series of adoption studies conducted in Scandinavia discussed earlier, as well as from replications in North American samples (D. W. Goodwin and Warnock 1991). In essence, the data show that adoptees with an alcoholic biological parent are much more likely to become alcoholic themselves.

Those with a liability to alcoholism are more likely to experience drinking alcohol as pleasurable, even upon the first exposure. They are therefore more likely to become dependent on the substance over time (Heath 1993). This finding is a good example of how genes influence both susceptibility to the environment and exposure to environmental risk factors.

In addition to a predisposition to alcoholism itself, another genetic mechanism may involve the transmission of impulsive personality traits. Thus, in a recent American adoption study (Cadoret et al. 1995a), antisocial personality in biological parents was associated with conduct disorder and drug abuse in their adopted-away children.

A somewhat different hypothesis was proposed many years ago by Winokur et al. (1969), who suggested that alcoholism could be sex-linked in its inheritance, with the same genetic predisposition expressing itself in females as somatization disorder. However, this theory was not supported by later research (D. W. Goodwin and Warnock 1991). In any case, it is unlikely that the genetic factors in alcoholism act through a single major gene. As in most psychiatric disorders, the hereditary influences on alcoholism are probably mediated through polygenic mechanisms.

Recently, large-scale research projects have been undertaken to discover specific gene linkages associated with a predisposition to alcoholism (Reich 1996). However, some of the initial attempts have not been successful. Thus, reports of an A1 allele linkage of the dopamine D_2 receptor (Blum et al. 1990) were not confirmed by other investigators (Bolos et al. 1990).

Alcoholism is another example of a disorder in which early onset is a marker for a stronger genetic predisposition. Thus, as reviewed earlier, evidence from adoption studies points to a stronger predisposition in type 2 alcoholism. In a large-scale study, Buydens-Branchey et al. (1989) also found that an onset of alcohol abuse before age 20 in men was associated with higher rates of paternal alcoholism.

The pattern of father-to-son transmission in alcoholism has been an important focus of recent research (Pihl and Peterson 1990). Thus, we can search for biological markers associated with susceptibility to alcoholism in this group. The sons of alcoholic men differ from control subjects in several ways: they have a much greater tolerance for alcohol, show differences in event-related potentials as measured by electroencephalography, and also demonstrate abnormalities on neuropsychological testing (Schuckit 1986).

Tarter et al. (1995) have reviewed studies examining the temperamental factors that place individuals at risk for alcoholism. These risk factors include higher behavioral activity, shorter attention span, higher harm avoidance, higher novelty seeking, and greater sociability. It should be noted that these traits are also associated with many other disorders, such as attention-deficit/hyperactivity disorder and antisocial personality disorder, which can often be comorbid with alcoholism.

Researchers are currently investigating whether some of these traits are linked to genetic markers (Benjamin et al. 1996).

D. W. Goodwin (1985) has suggested a theory in which alcohol is abused by those who have insufficient levels of endogenous brain chemicals. He proposed that alcohol has a biphasic action on the brain: it first corrects for a deficiency (possibly of serotonin, dopamine, or endorphins) but then creates an even greater deficiency, which leads to a craving for even more of the substance.

This model could explain why those who are most susceptible to abuse tend to be highly tolerant of alcohol, and why they enjoy their initial exposure to the substance. Individuals with a family history of alcoholism have increased endorphin sensitivity (Gianoulakis et al. 1996). The other side of this coin is that those who have an unpleasant reaction to alcohol are much less likely to become addicted (Schuckit and Smith 1996). One dysphoric reaction is the "oriental flush," an autonomic reaction more common in East Asian populations (D. W. Goodwin and Warnock 1991), which might partially explain the lower prevalence of alcoholism seen in some of these groups.

In summary, it is absolutely clear that a vulnerability to alcoholism is heritable. However, we do not know *what* is inherited. Individual differences in the effects of alcohol on the brain could be the effects of a specific predisposition or could depend on the presence of one or several personality traits. We also do not know whether these predispositions are specific to alcohol or are equally associated with an increased risk for abusing other substances.

Two aspects of alcoholism require particular attention: its relationship to mood disorders and its differential sex prevalence. One of the hypotheses about alcohol abuse has been that alcoholic individuals are really "treating" themselves for depression. Some research (e.g., Winokur et al. 1969) has indicated that alcoholism and depression can run in the same families, which suggests that the two conditions might represent different expressions of the same predisposition. One piece of evidence supporting this view is that among the Amish of Pennsylvania, a group in which alcoholism is extremely rare, the female preponderance for severe depression seen in most American populations is not found (Egeland and Hostetter 1976).

Any theory of the etiology of alcoholism must explain the large sex differences in its prevalence. As proposed in Chapter 2, diseases are more heritable in the gender in which they are less common. However, empirical findings remain contradictory: in an Australian twin study, Heath et al. (1997) found no gender differences in alcoholism prevalence, while in an adoption study, Cutrona et al. (1994) confirmed the strong genetic factors in the etiology of alcoholism in men, but found a larger environmental component in women.

Stressors

Some clinicians assume that the self-destructive behaviors associated with alcoholism must have their roots in an unhappy childhood. Retrospective studies in which patients are asked about their life experiences are likely to elicit such recollections. However, this method fails to separate the effects of genes and environment on substance abuse. Moreover, alcoholic patients are known for their tendency to blame others, not excluding their parents, for their current problems. Prospective research is needed in which childhood variables are measured prior to the onset of substance abuse.

Few studies have been conducted in which young children have been followed into adulthood to see whether they develop alcoholism. However, Masse and Tremblay (1996), following a cohort from kindergarten until adolescence, report that personality dimensions can be used to identify boys who are most likely to develop drinking problems later. Using Cloninger's "three dimensional" personality schema (see Chapter 15), these researchers found that the risk for alcoholism was associated with traits of high novelty seeking and low harm avoidance. Other research (Vaillant 1994) examined adolescents who had not yet developed alcoholism, first assessing their family backgrounds retrospectively and then following the cohort prospectively for many years. This study found that family history was a good predictor of later alcoholism but failed to show that the quality of childhood experience was related to addiction in adulthood. These results support the conclusion that predispositions are a necessary cause of alcoholism.

Although some individuals who subsequently develop alcoholism have behavioral problems in childhood and adolescence, most are asymptomatic prior to developing addiction. Moreover, when alcoholic individuals stop drinking, they do not necessarily show residual symptoms of other disorders (Vaillant 1994). If, on the other hand, they return to alcohol, the previous degree of behavioral psychopathology returns in all its severity (Vaillant 1996). These findings suggest that in those who are susceptible to substance abuse, psychopathology is often the *result* of the addiction rather than its cause.

The most important environmental factors mediating the expression of a predisposition to alcohol are social. Although no society has been described in which alcoholism is totally absent, there are striking differences in its prevalence in countries around the world (Helzer and Canino 1992). In a prospective study, Vaillant (1994) also noted that the prevalence varies a great deal among different ethnic groups in America.

Some of the cross-cultural differences in alcoholism might be accounted for by racial differences associated with genetically determined dysphoric physical effects experienced whenever alcohol is imbibed (D. W. Goodwin and Warnock 1991). However, such explanations cannot account for other cross-national differences, such as the high rate of alcoholism in France and the much lower rate in Italy. Most likely, social factors are responsible for these differences.

Genetic predispositions to alcoholism can be either suppressed or amplified by social attitudes toward drinking. These social factors include where people drink (e.g., in bars, at the dinner table) as well as whether heavy drinking is encouraged. We cannot explain the preponderance of male alcoholics entirely on the basis of predispositions. Consequently, it is probable that social factors in males influence their vulnerability, since in many societies, men drink to establish bonding, whereas women do not.

In summary, a combination of genetic predisposition, substance exposure, and social reinforcement accounts for the development of alcoholism in men. Women, in whom alcohol is much more likely to be used as self-medication, probably have a different pathway to alcohol abuse.

Similar principles may apply to other forms of substance abuse. Future research should help to clarify in more detail whether the same mechanisms are involved in drug addiction. A recent study of heredity and environment in cannabis use (Kendler and Prescott 1998) supports this idea. In adoption studies (e.g., Cadoret et al. 1986), abuse of many different drugs is more likely in individuals who have a biological parent diagnosed with either alcoholism or antisocial personality disorder.

Substance abuse has also been found to be associated with a number of psychosocial risk factors, such as an impoverished urban background, parental separation, and a dysfunctional family structure (Haastrup and Thomsen 1972; Helzer et al. 1976). None of these risk factors necessarily leads to the abuse of substances, since only those who are predisposed will develop addictions.

▇ Summary: Predisposition and Stress in Substance Abuse

Substance abuse provides one of the best-documented examples of the predisposition–stress model in psychopathology. The research evidence shows that there are genetic predispositions to alcoholism, and that social factors strongly influence the prevalence of abuse. Future investigations will probably support a similar model for other forms of substance abuse.

The most parsimonious explanation of the data on alcoholism is as follows:

1. Individuals with the strongest predisposition to alcoholism may develop the disorder in any cultural setting where the substance is available.
2. When the culture encourages excessive drinking, those with weaker predispositions will also be affected, and alcoholism will be more common.
3. If the culture discourages excessive drinking, those with weaker predispositions will not abuse alcohol, and alcoholism will be less common.

13

Eating Disorders

The two categories of eating disorder, anorexia nervosa and bulimia nervosa, manifest quite different symptoms. Anorexic individuals restrict their eating, whereas bulimic individuals lose control of their intake. However, both disorders derive from interactions between genetic predispositions and psychosocial stressors.

Anorexia nervosa and bulimia nervosa overlap in some cases, so that anorexic patients with binges are more like patients with bulimia than like those with typical anorexia (Steiger and Stotland 1995). Moreover, anorexia nervosa and bulimia nervosa are themselves heterogeneous disorders, with severe cases deriving from different etiological pathways than milder cases.

Some years ago, Garner et al. (1984) hypothesized two components in the eating disorders: a specific factor concerning weight control and body image, and nonspecific factors associated with a general predisposition to psychopathology. Many people worry about their weight, but few ever develop eating disorders. Other risk factors determine whether attitudes about body image are normal or pathological. Thus, weight control may not become a serious problem unless other predispositions are also present.

Predispositions to Anorexia Nervosa

Anorexia nervosa can be a life-threatening disease. As with other mental disorders, we would expect that the more severe an illness is, the more likely it is to involve a strong genetic predisposition. The evidence supports this expectation.

A British twin study by Holland et al. (1988) found a strong genetic predisposition to anorexia nervosa, with a concordance of 55% in monozygotic (MZ) twins but only 7% in dizygotic (DZ) twins. In a later replication by the same research group (Treasure and Holland 1995), the differences were somewhat less striking but still significant, with an MZ concordance of 65% and a DZ concordance of 32%. Treasure and Holland (1995) also examined those MZ pairs that were not concordant for anorexia nervosa and found that they had a later age at onset of illness.

Obesity is not unusually frequent among the relatives of anorexic patients (Treasure and Holland 1995). This finding is in accord with the fact that instead of being prone to weight gain, most anorexic patients are "restrictors" in their eating behavior. It is also not surprising that these traits are associated with comorbidity for personality disorders in the anxious cluster (Steiger and Stotland 1995; Steiger et al. 1996). Moreover, community studies (Rastam and Gillberg 1991) as well as twin studies (Treasure and Holland 1995) have found that the genetic predisposition to anorexia nervosa is strongly associated with compulsive personality traits, particularly traits of perfectionism. Rastam (1992) has even suggested that anorexia nervosa is a type of compulsive symptom.

Predispositions to Bulimia Nervosa

Bulimia nervosa is a much less severe illness than anorexia. Its boundaries with abnormal eating behavior are fuzzy (Garfinkel et al. 1995), and it is much more prevalent than anorexia. We would therefore expect bulimia to have a strong environmental component.

Research findings tend to confirm these expectations (Treasure and Holland 1995). Two twin studies (Fichter and Noegel 1990; Hsu et al. 1990) drawn from clinical samples supported a heritable predisposition to bulimia nervosa, but in a larger sample, Treasure and Holland (1995) found no evidence for heritability. In a large-scale community twin study, Kendler et al. (1991) also found no differences between MZ and DZ concordance for bulimic symptoms. The overall conclusion is that the genetic factors in bulimia nervosa seem to be weak.

These contradictions reflect the heterogeneity of bulimia nervosa, an illness that has become very common. Its etiology involves strong psychosocial factors; thus, bulimia nervosa can develop in the absence of any strong predisposition, although the more severe cases that appear in clinical samples may depend more on genetic factors.

There are three types of predispositions to bulimia nervosa: 1) a tendency to become obese, 2) impulsive personality traits, and 3) a susceptibility to depression.

Although not present in all cases, there is a strong association between a predisposition to develop bulimia nervosa and a tendency to become overweight. Obesity is unusually common among the relatives of patients with bulimia nervosa (Treasure and Holland 1995); thus, it follows that bulimic patients are trying to maintain their weight below a natural "set point" (Garner and Garfinkel 1985). We should therefore examine the nature of the predisposition to obesity itself.

Some people have constant trouble maintaining their weight, while others remain svelte without difficulty. In an adoption study, Stunkard et al. (1986) found that the tendency to obesity is strongly heritable. In a Darwinian context, this should not be surprising. A trait favoring fat storage would have been very useful in the environment in which our species evolved. Although those who stayed thin would be generally healthier under normal conditions, those with a genetic tendency to obesity would have a greater capacity to store calories and would therefore be better protected against inevitable food shortages (Nesse and Williams 1994). These genetic variations would not have caused obesity in environments in which there was little excess food to be eaten and in which regular exercise was a necessity for survival rather than simply an elective health-promoting activity.

In modern societies, in which food is abundant and exercise can be avoided, there are bound to be more obese individuals. It is the social pressure to be thin, particularly among women, that leads many people to make serious efforts to lose weight. Excessive dieting is, in fact, often a major triggering factor in bulimia nervosa (Polivy and Herman 1985).

However, since only a few dieters ever develop bingeing and purging, this factor does not fully explain the development of bulimic symptoms.

The second element in the predisposition to develop eating disorders involves personality traits. Personality structures among bulimic individuals are variable, although traits of impulsivity and novelty seeking are common (Steiger et al. 1996). In bulimia nervosa, patients try to restrict their eating but are unable to do so. Their symptoms then become the opposite of the restriction seen in anorexia nervosa, with a loss of control and an inability to stop a binge once it starts. In this respect, bulimia nervosa resembles other addictive disorders, such as substance abuse. There is considerable comorbidity of bulimia with substance abuse (Halmi 1994). Moreover, both bulimia nervosa and substance abuse are comorbid with impulsive personality disorders (Halmi 1994). The more severe the bulimia, the more likely the patient is to have Axis II comorbidity in the impulsive cluster, usually in either the histrionic or the borderline category (Steiger et al. 1991; Vitousek and Manke 1994). These observations point to impulsivity as an essential element in the development of bulimia nervosa.

Impulsivity as a trait is related to reduced serotonergic activity (Siever and Davis 1991). Some studies have suggested that bulimic patients have a sluggish serotonergic system (Goldbloom and Garfinkel 1990). Clinical trials also show that specific serotonin reuptake inhibitors are useful in controlling binges, and this effect, since it requires very high doses, is more likely to be based on reduced impulsivity than on antidepressant activity (Goldbloom and Garfinkel 1990).

Finally, some bulimic patients also have a predisposition to mood disorders, as indicated by their family histories (Steiger and Stotland 1995). It seems likely that in many cases, overeating functions as a mechanism to suppress depressive dysphoria.

Psychological Factors in Eating Disorders

In both anorexia nervosa and bulimia nervosa, psychological stressors lowering self-esteem lead individuals to focus on their weight as a representation of their personal worth. However, no specific life experiences are associated with either of these conditions.

The most extensive study of the psychological background of anorexic patients was conducted in Gôteborg, Sweden (Rastam 1992; Rastam and Gillberg 1991). This study examined 51 anorexic patients drawn from a population sample rather than from clinical settings. No "typical" family structure was associated with anorexia nervosa. Rastam's group did not confirm the hypothesis of Minuchin et al. (1978) that anorexic families are unusually rigid and enmeshed. The authors concluded that factors intrinsic to the patient are much more important than family structure in anorexia nervosa.

As we have seen in depression and substance abuse, there is no clear boundary between bulimia nervosa and abnormal eating behavior. A genetic epidemiological study by Kendler et al. (1991) showed that the risk factors for "narrowly defined bulimia nervosa" and for "bulimia nervosa–like syndromes" are very similar. These included a history of weight fluctuation, dieting or frequent exercise, and a slim ideal body image. Kendler's data were consistent with a multiple-threshold model, with one threshold for a more severe form of pathology (narrowly defined bulimia nervosa) and another for less severe forms (bulimia nervosa–like syndromes).

As reviewed by Steiger and Stotland (1995), the most consistent findings in the literature concerning bulimia nervosa describe families that are high in conflict, low in cohesion, and low in emotional responsiveness. However, this picture is not very specific to bulimia; similar family characteristics can be found in a variety of other diagnoses. Moreover, developmental adversities in bulimic patients are strongly related to Axis II comorbidity (Steiger et al. 1996). As Steiger and Stotland (1995) conclude, studies of the psychological risks for bulimia nervosa "inform us more about the way in which many forms of psychopathology represent a collision between social pressures and psychological vulnerabilities than about the development of eating disorders per se" (p. 63).

■ Social Factors: Eating Disorders as Culture-Bound Syndromes

In an apocryphal story, the Duchess of Windsor is said to have remarked, "a woman can never be too rich or too thin." Social factors, by encouraging people to seek unrealistic levels of slimness, lower the threshold for excessive concerns about body image. These social factors are particularly strong in North American and European societies. One has only to browse through any bookstore to appreciate how important dieting has become in our culture. These social pressures are much more common in the upper classes, whereas overt obesity is more common in lower socioeconomic groups (Steiger and Stotland 1995).

These considerations also help to explain why eating disorders, as common as they are in modern social structures, are rarely seen in traditional societies. This situation is changing as cultures around the globe undergo modernization. For example, eating disorders have been diagnosed for the first time in the children of immigrants in economically developed countries (e.g., families moving from Southern to Northern Europe) (DiNicola 1990). We have also seen a striking increase in the prevalence of eating disorders in our own society (Halmi 1994; Jones et al. 1980). Moreover, in economically developed countries, high rates of eating disorders have spread from upper to lower socioeconomic levels (Steiger and Stotland 1995).

Diagnoses that exist only in specific cultural settings can be thought of, at least from our own perspective, as "exotic." However, the findings just described show that eating disorders can readily be classified with those psychiatric entities that transcultural psychiatrists (Murphy 1982) term "culture-bound syndromes," reflecting the cultural molding of universal vulnerabilities (Prince and Tseng-Laroche 1990).

The best explanation for the increased prevalence of eating disorders in modern societies is that these disorders derive from a culturally shaped pursuit of thinness (Garner and Garfinkel 1985). Thinness is rarely a goal in cultures that have known starvation or high levels of mortality in children, and in which children are consequently seen as healthier when they are slightly overweight.

On the other hand, in economically developed countries, in which hunger is unknown and children rarely die, milder degrees of obesity may be seen by young females as reducing their sexual attractiveness. This gender difference reflects a biological given, the greater importance of physical beauty in women (Buss 1994). In this context, the overwhelmingly higher prevalence of eating disorders in women should not be very surprising.

The first clinical description of anorexia nervosa (Gull 1873) was published in the 19th century. Fairly typical cases can be identified from the medical literature at that period (Brumberg 1988). Prior to that time, the structure of European societies resembled in most ways that of societies that remain economically underdeveloped today. Therefore, concerns with body image were probably much less common then. As documented by historians (Brumberg 1988; Vanderveycken and van Deth 1994), cases of self-starvation prior to the 19th century were usually related to excessive religious preoccupations.

Social Factors: Sociocultural Risks for Eating Disorders

That cultural factors play a crucial role in eating disorders is supported by the lack of any clear boundaries between pathological and normal attitudes toward eating. Studies using a self-report instrument, the Eating Attitudes Test (EAT; Garner and Garfinkel 1979), in nonclinical populations found no clear cutoff between dysfunctional eating attitudes and diagnosable eating disorders (Garfinkel et al. 1995).

What are the reasons for the pervasive pursuit of thinness among women in developed countries? Evolutionary psychology can shed some light on this question. Among fertile women, selection favors those who shape their behaviors to compete most successfully for partners (Buss 1994). Darwinian theory (Cronin 1991) describes two types of selection: *natural selection,* which depends on survival and reproduction, and *sexual selection,* which can be contrary to survival in the long run but favorable in the short run because the trait in question increases the likelihood of finding a mate.

The cult of female beauty is an example of both kinds of selection. From the point of view of natural selection, the characteristics that define female beauty in all cultures are markers for fertility (Buss 1994). Thus, men tend to look for signs of youth and good health in a potential mate. From the point of view of sexual selection, beauty is an exaggerated characteristic that often serves no useful function except for the crucial one of attracting a mate.

Slimness is a marker for youth and fertility. However, like the tail of the peacock, exaggerated thinness does not necessarily imply better health. Evolutionary psychologists refer to a "supernormal stimulus," i.e., a trait exaggerated by sexual selection (Cronin 1991). Such stimuli can become more valued when other elements in the assessment of body type—i.e., those that are crucial to health—are less important.

In a society in which food is scarce, female beauty assumes less importance. A farmer might be more interested in strength than slimness in a wife. However, under conditions of abundance, sexual preferences of men for slimmer women are more likely to become exaggerated. The pursuit of thinness and beauty is further exaggerated by the influences of fashion and advertising. Models have always been chosen to be unusually thin, and when Garner and Garfinkel (1980) examined centerfolds of *Playboy* magazine over several decades, they found a steadily increasing preference for thinness.

Traditional societies reduce the intensity of sexual selection. These cultures provide mates (albeit not always the most desirable ones) for virtually anyone who wishes to be married. In modern societies, in contrast, women have excellent reasons to fear not being able to find a partner and thus not being able to reproduce.

It is only in developed societies that we see socioeconomic differences in the prevalence of eating disorders (more common in the upper classes) and obesity (more common in the lower classes) (Halmi 1994). In other words, although many women in developed societies are tempted to overeat, those in the lower classes suffer less consequences if they do, whereas those in the upper classes have more practical reasons to overcome their urges, leading to a greater concern with dieting.

These sociocultural factors affect everyone in our society. However, patients with eating disorders, particularly those with bulimia nervosa, are especially susceptible to these cultural influences.

■ Summary: Gene–Environment Interactions in Eating Disorders

Several authors (Johnson and Connors 1987; Steiger and Stotland 1995) have suggested a multidimensional perspective on eating disorders that is essentially identical to a predisposition–stress model.

The evidence indicates that anorexic individuals show the following:

- a strong genetic predisposition
- compulsive and perfectionistic personality traits
- restriction of eating to obtain control over their bodies

In contrast, bulimic individuals demonstrate the following:

- a greater vulnerability to environmental factors
- impulsive personality traits
- a natural set point that tends to make them slightly overweight
- a stronger response to the cultural pursuit of thinness

In summary, anorexia nervosa and bulimia nervosa are complex disorders that develop in the presence of a combination of biological predispositions, psychological stressors, and powerful social influences.

14

Disorders Arising in Childhood

An early age at onset of illness is often a marker for biological vulnerability. It should therefore not be surprising that many of the most frequent disorders arising in childhood involve genetic predispositions.

Child psychiatric disorders with an obvious organic component, including many forms of mental retardation, learning disorders, and communication disorders, all show a strong hereditary component (Rutter et al. 1990). However, in the present chapter, we will focus on three disorders beginning in childhood that have not always been recognized to involve genetic predispositions. Each of these has now been sufficiently well researched to demonstrate the relationships between nature and nurture in their development. In *attention-deficit disorder,* genetic predispositions are strong but require activation by environmental stressors. In *conduct disorder,* environmental factors are crucial, but predispositions play a role in more severe cases. Finally, *autistic disorder* is a condition that was once thought to be environmental but is now known to be strongly heritable.

Attention-Deficit/Hyperactivity Disorder

Boundaries

Attention-deficit/hyperactivity disorder (ADHD) has a prevalence of between 5% and 10% in boys, and of between 2% and 4% in girls (Wender
1987). These rates, particularly for males, are high—much higher, indeed, than those for most adult psychiatric disorders (with the notable
exception of alcoholism). Such a high prevalence suggests that we are
looking at a widely distributed trait that only sometimes presents as a
mental disorder.

The diagnostic construct of ADHD defined in DSM-IV (American
Psychiatric Association 1994) has two components: 1) a deficit in maintaining attention and 2) an abnormal level of activity and impulsivity.
Different patients may show a predominance of one or the other of
these problems. Of the two, increased activity associated with impulsivity is the most likely to bring children to clinical attention and is the
most disabling aspect of the condition. Since boys are usually more
physically active than girls, it is not surprising that attention-deficit disorder with hyperactivity is more common in males, while attention-
deficit disorder without hyperactivity has a relatively equal sex distribution (G. Weiss and Hechtman 1992).

There is a lower threshold for the diagnosis of ADHD in North America than in Britain, where attention-deficit disorder is less commonly diagnosed, largely because it is seen as secondary to conduct disorder
(C. W. Popper and Steingard 1994). ADHD with hyperactivity is highly
comorbid with conduct disorder, and it is those children with both
diagnoses who are most often referred for assessment (Rutter 1985).
When ADHD is not accompanied by conduct disorder, as is more often
the case among girls, it may not be detected clinically, even though it
may cause problems with academic performance.

Although ADHD begins in childhood, it does not always "burn out"
over time. Follow-up studies show that individuals with ADHD in
childhood may continue to have symptoms in adulthood, and that
about one-fifth of ADHD children, particularly those with comorbid
conduct disorder, will develop antisocial personality disorder (Manuzza et al. 1998; G. Weiss and Hechtman 1992). As a result of these

findings, there has been a great deal of interest in diagnosing and treating previously unrecognized ADHD in adult populations.

Attention-deficit disorder in adults also has a high comorbidity with mood disorders and personality disorders (Biederman et al. 1996). In view of these associations, Shaffer (1994) has cautioned psychiatrists against being too eager to make the "fashionable" diagnosis of adult ADHD. Many cases that meet DSM criteria might be better understood as reflecting depression and/or Axis II pathology.

These findings raise questions about the boundaries of ADHD. At what point do problems in attention, activity, and impulsivity cause sufficient dysfunction to be called psychopathological? Can we separate ADHD from the other diagnoses with which it is comorbid? The predisposition–stress model may help shed light on these questions.

Predispositions

Twin studies have consistently reported significant differences in monozygotic–dizygotic concordance for ADHD (Hechtman 1994; Levy et al. 1997; Rutter et al. 1997; Silberg et al. 1996). An adoption study (Cadoret and Stewart 1991) has also confirmed these findings. Whether ADHD and conduct disorders are independent of each other remains uncertain. One large-scale family study (Biederman et al. 1992; Faraone et al. 1991) has reported strong familial patterns for ADHD that were independent of the disorder's comorbidity, but a twin study by Silberg et al. (1996) found genetic variance common to both ADHD and conduct disorder. No definite mode of inheritance has emerged from these genetic studies.

The predisposition to ADHD can also be seen in genetic studies of the disorder's underlying traits. Stevenson (1992), in a population-based twin study, found that activity levels in healthy children have a heritability of 75%. It would be interesting to see whether similar findings apply to attentional levels.

Biological markers would be useful to make the diagnosis of ADHD more precise. Hyperactive children show a number of neuropsychological abnormalities, and neuroimaging studies have suggested that these children may have functional abnormalities in brain activity (Hechtman 1994). However, the precise pathophysiology behind ADHD is not known.

Most mental disorders arising in childhood are more common in males. Chapter 2 discussed the principle that gender differences in prevalence are usually associated with a greater genetic penetrance in the less frequently affected sex. The disorders arising in childhood largely confirm these expectations, in that we see stronger environmental factors in boys and stronger genetic factors in girls (McGuffin and Gottesman 1985). These differences apply to ADHD, in which girls frequently have a stronger family history of the disorder than do boys (Vandenberg et al. 1986).

ADHD is also an example of the relationship between age at onset and heritability. The more familial a case of ADHD, the earlier its onset and the more likely it is to continue into adulthood (Biederman et al. 1996). Moreover, the offspring of adults with ADHD are more likely to develop the disorder (Biederman et al. 1995a). These findings suggest that ADHD cases that start early and continue into adulthood involve a stronger genetic component, whereas later-onset cases that "burn out" early may be more environmental in origin. (Later in this chapter, we will observe a similar pattern for conduct disorder.)

Stressors

Although ADHD has a strong biological basis, environmental factors may be a necessary condition for the emergence of the disorder. As reviewed by Campbell (1990), several psychosocial risk factors tend to be associated with ADHD: family conflict, parental psychopathology, and indicators of social adversity. None of these are specific to ADHD. In fact, they are the general risk factors for psychopathology in children, associated with a variety of clinical diagnoses. Although psychopathology in children can increase levels of family conflict, it is unlikely that these risk factors are merely parental responses to children with abnormal temperaments.

The environmental factors in disorders of childhood depend on the cumulative effects of multiple risks. In a classic epidemiological study, Rutter et al. (1975) examined a series of measures of adversity, which, in concert, significantly raised the risk for the development of any psychiatric diagnosis in children. These indicators were severe marital discord, low social class, large family size, paternal criminality, maternal mental disorder, and foster care placement. Scores on a scale measuring all of these factors were better predictors than was any single factor of the development of psychiatric disorders of all types. Biederman et al. (1995b) have used Rutter's scale to determine the environmental risk factors for ADHD. They found that the more of these indicators were present, the more likely children were to develop this disorder. Yet, the same risk factors also predict the development of other "externalizing" disorders (e.g., conduct disorder), as well as of "internalizing" disorders (e.g., depression, anxiety).

Gene–Environment Interactions

The high prevalence of ADHD in males points to the presence of a widely distributed predisposition interacting with prevalent psychosocial stressors. The mechanisms may be similar to those described for nonmelancholic unipolar depression in Chapter 9, for alcoholism in Chapter 12, and for bulimia nervosa in Chapter 13.

Essentially, the following argument could account for much of the data. Attentional capacity and activity–impulsivity levels are intercorrelated traits that are continuously distributed in the population. At some threshold, low attention and high activity are more likely to become problematic. This threshold is influenced by the strength of predispositions, but is also dependent on the nature of stressors. The most important environmental precipitants are the demands of a classroom and the presence of family dysfunction.

The presence of a coexisting conduct disorder, which so often brings ADHD children to clinical attention, can be thought of as a marker for the environmental factors associated with that diagnosis, most particularly the failure of parents to supervise and discipline their children effectively. As we will see later in this chapter, conduct disorder, which is even more heterogeneous than ADHD, depends on stronger environmental factors.

ADHD, in spite of its roots in biological variability, should therefore show large differences in its prevalence across cultures and across social contexts. We have already noted that the disorder is diagnosed much less frequently in Britain. These transatlantic differences could have several explanations. The North American criteria for ADHD could be too broad. Alternatively, British psychiatrists could be missing ADHD because they concentrate too much on comorbid conduct disorder. Finally, higher levels of discipline in British schools might suppress the symptoms of ADHD. There is a clear need for transcultural studies of ADHD to sort out these possibilities.

ADHD probably derives from a widely distributed trait that need not, in and of itself, be dysfunctional. Every trait has to be understood in terms of its original function in the environment in which our species evolved. In hunter–gatherer and agrarian societies, men with a shorter attention span and higher levels of activity–impulsivity might have actually functioned better in settings where overt aggression and rapid responses were useful for survival. However, in a modern society, interactions between these traits and specific social demands, such as the expectation that young boys sit down and pay attention in a classroom, can cause trouble.

There are no biological advantages to sitting quietly in class, to listening to a teacher, or to reading a book. Rather, these sociocultural expectations have developed only in modern societies. As recently as a few generations ago, children who could not cope with these expectations could leave school at an early age and go to work. It is interesting in this regard that ADHD was first described in the medical literature about 100 years ago (Still 1902), around the same time that child labor was being abolished.

Many patients with ADHD never present clinically in childhood. These individuals may be able to work around their problems with attention, activity, and impulsivity, at least until a major psychosocial stressor or the cumulative demands of work and family responsibilities overwhelm their compensatory mechanisms (Hechtman 1994).

In about 20% of boys with ADHD, the disorder is a precursor of antisocial personality disorder in adulthood (G. Weiss and Hechtman 1992). One of the strongest correlates of this outcome is the presence of externalizing disorders in parents (Herrero et al. 1992). As we will see in the next section, parental pathology is also crucial in predicting whether children with conduct disorder go on to become antisocial adults.

In summary, children with ADHD are a heterogeneous population. Many children have strong biological predispositions associated with an early onset and a chronic course of illness. Others have weaker predispositions that become amplified to dysfunctional levels only when they are exposed to major environmental stressors.

Conduct Disorder

Conduct disorder (CD), like ADHD, is a very high-prevalence disorder, affecting between 5% and 10% of boys and about 2%–3% of girls (Martin and Hoffman 1990). One-third of children with CD go on to develop antisocial personality disorder (L. N. Robins 1966). This outcome is more likely when there are more symptoms, when symptoms are severe, and when symptoms have an early onset (Martin and Hoffman 1990; Zoccolillo et al. 1992). Moreover, conduct disorder can also be a precursor of other forms of psychopathology, ranging from mood disorder to psychosis (Zoccolillo 1992)

Conduct disorder is unlike most of the other forms of psychopathology that arise in childhood in that most empirical research suggests that the symptoms of CD are *not* strongly heritable. Moreover, unlike the environmental factors in other psychiatric disorders in children, those in CD tend to be *shared* (i.e., derived from living in the same family) rather than unshared (i.e., derived from factors outside the family) (Pike and Plomin 1996; Rutter et al. 1997). Thus, conduct problems often reflect the effects of a pathogenic family environment.

The criteria for conduct disorder involve behaviors that violate the basic rights of others. An abnormal level of aggressiveness as a trait may lie behind these overt behaviors. Behavioral genetic studies in community populations show that aggressivity is unlike most other personality traits, in that it involves a negligible genetic component, with most of the environmental factors in aggression being shared (Martin and Hoffman 1990).

Lyons et al. (1995) examined the concordance between juvenile and adult antisocial traits in a large twin registry and found that such traits predicted adult pathology when they were present during adolescence but *not* when they occurred in childhood. Moreover, in this study, the shared environment accounted for 31% of conduct symptoms. A longitudinal study of twins (Rutter et al. 1997) has also reported that genetic factors are relatively weak in conduct disorder, except in cases where symptoms persist into adulthood. The only dissenting findings, from a recent Australian twin study (Slutske et al. 1997), were limited by that study's use of a retrospective methodology.

We can conclude that conduct disorder is, in the largest number of cases, an outcome of defective parenting. The most likely mechanism, as shown by a large body of research (Martin and Hoffman 1990), involves the failure to provide children with discipline in a consistent fashion.

However, conduct disorder is heterogeneous. Even though most children with conduct disorder are responding to environmental stressors, a subgroup of children who go on to exhibit adult antisocial behavior have stronger genetic predispositions (Lyons 1996; Lyons et al. 1995). These predispositions may involve impulsive personality traits (see Chapter 15). One line of evidence for this hypothesis emerges from a longitudinal follow-up comparing the development of infants with different temperaments (Schwartz et al. 1996). When aggressive ("uninhibited") versus nonaggressive ("inhibited") children are followed into adolescence, the first group is much more likely to develop conduct disorder (Kerr et al. 1997). When these temperamental differences can be observed very early in life and are severe, they provide a strong basis to predict that symptoms will continue into adulthood (Zoccolillo et al. 1992).

A second line of evidence supporting the importance of temperament in this subgroup of conduct disorder is that adopted children as a group are somewhat more likely to develop impulsive symptoms (Bohman and Sigvardsson 1980). A likely explanation is that the parents who give up their children for adoption tend to have more impulsive character traits. Moreover, conduct disorder is more frequent in children whose biological mothers have antisocial traits (Bohman and Sigvardsson 1980). Antisocial traits were found to be more heritable in females, and given the lower rate of antisocial personality in women, females with delinquency may have a greater genetic component.

These studies also help to elucidate the role of environmental factors in conduct disorder. Thus, Cadoret et al. (1995b) showed that even for adoptees with an antisocial biological parent, children developed symptoms only if they also experienced an adverse adoptive home environment. Moreover, parental pathology accounted for much less of the variance in childhood symptoms than in adolescent or adult symptoms.

Essentially, children who go on to develop adult criminality are a different group from those who do not. Only the subgroup of children who go on to develop antisocial personality have strong predispositions. Genetic factors have been shown to be much stronger for adult criminality than for childhood delinquency (Rutter 1989; Rutter and Maughan 1997). The majority of children with conduct disorder outgrow their delinquent behaviors because they lack these genetic predispositions. Instead, these children are responding to a stressful environment from which they can eventually escape.

The environmental predictors of CD are essentially those described by Rutter et al. (1975) as adversities leading to most forms of psychopathology in children. They include severe marital discord, low social class, large family size, paternal criminality, maternal mental disorder, and foster care placement. Research over the last two decades confirms the importance of these risk factors. For example, in one recent prospective study, the strongest correlates of conduct disorder were parental substance abuse and low socioeconomic status (Loeber et al. 1995).

In summary, research findings are consistent with the following model:

1. Children with conduct disorder are heterogeneous, with most having no specific genetic liability, and with symptoms being precipitated primarily by family dysfunction.
2. Genetic factors are more important in individuals with early and more severe symptoms and in those who go on to develop antisocial personality disorder.
3. Even when genetic factors predispose an individual to conduct disorder, these effects emerge only in the presence of interactions with family pathology.

■ Autistic Disorder: A Cautionary Tale

Autistic disorder, unlike ADHD and CD, is a rare disease. It is much more common in boys and affects only about 0.05% of the general population (Rutter 1991). Theories about its etiology have followed a historical trajectory somewhat similar to that described for schizophrenia in Chapter 8.

This condition was first described by Kanner (1943), who termed it "early infantile autism." Although Kanner thought that autism was probably constitutional, he also noted the presence of unusual problems in bonding between mother and child. In an era in which any problems with mothers in early childhood could be invoked to explain the origins of severe forms of psychopathology, Kanner's observation was interpreted as suggesting that autism developed *as a result of* this failure to bond. Instead of understanding a mother's emotional detachment from her autistic child as a reaction to the child's constitutional inability to attach, environmentalists assumed that the mother's behavior caused the child's pathology.

The apogee of environmental models of autism can be found in a book published by Bruno Bettelheim (1967), an analyst well known at the time for his work with severely disturbed children. Bettelheim argued that autism was a *defense* against a grossly defective and neglectful maternal environment. The reader will note, of course, the similarity of this formulation to analytic theories of schizophrenia. Ironically, Bettelheim was constructing his theory at the very moment that genetic and biological findings were about to refute it.

A large amount of research over the last 30 years (Folstein and Piven 1991) has demonstrated that autistic disorder has a strong genetic component. Rutter (1991) reported a heritability of 93%, much higher than that for bipolar mood disorder. (This may, however, be an overestimate, since the study from which the figure was derived had a monozygotic concordance of only 36%, and the dizygotic concordance was 0%; when such numbers are plugged into the heritability calculation, the final percentage comes out very high indeed.)

Autism may be an extreme outcome related to interactions of environmental factors with a trait that usually leads to subclinical abnormalities (Piven et al. 1997). The environmental components in autism, like those in schizophrenia, may unleash the disorder through mechanisms involving brain injury (Rutter 1991). The specific nature of these hypothesized brain lesions remains unknown.

As C. W. Popper and Steingard (1994) have stated, "there is no evidence that psychosocial factors or parenting abnormalities cause autistic disorder." The evolution of etiological models of autistic disorder is a cautionary tale because environmentalists, driven by their preconceptions about the importance of mothering, came to dramatically incorrect conclusions. Moreover, like the mothers of schizophrenic individuals, a generation of mothers unfortunate enough to have an autistic child were held unfairly accountable by psychiatrists for their children's plight.

The Predisposition–Stress Model in Child Psychiatry

At this point, we can underline some of the important interactions between predisposition and stress in the disorders arising in childhood.

1. There is no clear cutoff between normality and pathology. In particular, there is no sharp boundary between either hyperactivity or conduct disorder and underlying traits.
2. Disorders that arise early in life and that then become chronic have a stronger genetic component than those that appear for the first time later in life. This principle applies to early-onset ADHD, to the more severe cases of CD, and to autism.
3. Disorders that are more common in one sex tend to be based on stronger genetic factors when they appear in the opposite sex. This is the case for both ADHD and CD.
4. Each of the disorders arising in childhood has a different weighting of nature and nurture. In ADHD, environmental risk factors play an important but secondary role, while in CD, they are predominant in most cases. In autism, the environmental risk factors are probably biological.

Finally, the child development literature provides very little empirical support for the belief that adult mental disorders have their origins in childhood experiences. In fact, one of the most interesting things about the disorders arising in childhood are their *discontinuities* with adult mental disorders. Many children "grow out" of psychopathology. Although there are many exceptions to this principle, it applies to the two high-prevalence disorders discussed here: ADHD and CD. In fact, many if not most children with psychiatric disorders are never seen in adult clinics (Zeitlin 1986). Moreover, discontinuities are also found in the other direction: most adults with psychiatric disorders never had serious symptoms as children. These facts provide still another reason for clinicians to be cautious about accepting models that attempt to reduce all present problems to past experiences.

15

Personality Disorders

Personality disorders are an interesting example of the interactions between nature and nurture. In the past, many theorists assumed that biological factors played little role in personality development, that abnormal personality structures were largely environmental in origin, and that the stability of personality was explained by its roots in early childhood experience. The present chapter will show that all of these views are mistaken.

The most useful model of personality disorders views them as pathological exaggerations of normal personality traits. The pathways from traits to disorders would depend on both the strength of predispositions and the intensity of stressors. Individual differences in traits would correspond to the biological vulnerability for these disorders and determine the form that they take. Although temperamental differences must play some role in the predisposition to developing personality pathology, the most important factors determining whether or not traits actually develop into disorders may still be environmental (Nigg and Goldsmith 1998).

Personality Traits

Each individual has a unique way of responding to environmental challenges. These characteristics constitute what is commonly called "personality."

We can define personality *traits* as patterns of behavior, emotion, and cognition that remain consistent from one situation to another (Rutter 1987b). Traits show a great deal of variability among individuals. These characteristics can be identified early in life and tend to remain stable over a lifetime (Costa and McRae 1988).

Several schemata have been developed to describe personality traits or, as they are also called, personality *dimensions*. Most of these systems are derived from data drawn from self-report measures. Through the method of factor analysis, these questionnaire items can be grouped into psychological tests.

Some classifications have *broad* dimensions derived from the study of variability in normal personality. These dimensions describe basic characteristics such as *extraversion* (variations in the need for interpersonal contact) or *neuroticism* (variations in emotional stability)—two terms whose use dates back to the work of Jung (1921). In a highly influential schema, Eysenck (1991) developed these two dimensions, operationalized them, and placed them in a theoretical framework. (Eysenck later added a third basic dimension, *psychoticism*.)

Costa and McRae (1988) developed a model that adds three dimensions to Eysenck's original two. This Five-Factor Model consists of *extraversion–introversion, neuroticism, agreeableness, openness to experience,* and *conscientiousness*. Costa and Widiger (1994) have shown that these dimensions can usefully describe normal personality and can also account for most of the symptoms seen in personality disorder patients.

Cloninger (1987) focused on three dimensions of temperament: *novelty seeking, harm avoidance,* and *reward dependence*. More recently, Cloninger et al. (1993) added another temperamental dimension, *persistence*, as well as three "character dimensions."

Classifications that begin by describing psychopathology instead of normality tend to capture much more *narrow* dimensions of personality. Such schemata therefore require a much larger number of traits. Two of the classifications most widely used in research are Livesley et al.'s (1993) 18-dimensional schema and Tyrer's (1988) 24-dimensional schema.

The Origins of Personality

Both genetic and environmental factors play a role in the formation of adult personality. Traits are shaped during development by interactions between *temperament* and *social learning* (Rutter 1987b).

Temperament denotes behavioral dispositions present at birth. For example, infants can be more or less active, more or less socially responsive, more or less fearful, and more or less irritable. Within normal ranges, these variations in infantile temperament are not notably continuous with later personality traits (Chess and Thomas 1990). However, extreme temperaments are stronger predictors of pathology (Kagan 1994; Maziade et al. 1990). Infants who are extremely irritable or extremely fearful are likely to remain so, and these abnormal temperaments place them at risk for many problematic behaviors later in childhood. Temperamental effects are also not limited to characteristics present at birth, since some genetic effects may "switch on" only at later periods of development. This principle is demonstrated by the paradoxical observation that identical twins become more—not less—similar with age (see discussion in Rutter and Rutter 1993).

Temperament describes the heritable component of personality. Twin studies show that for most traits, whether broadly or narrowly defined, nearly 50% of the variance between individuals depends on genetic influences (Jang et al. 1996; Livesley et al. 1993; Plomin et al. 1990a). Moreover, monozygotic twins raised apart show striking similarities in their personality traits (Tellegen et al. 1988).

The fact that some traits are more influenced by environmental factors than others could be good news for the clinicians who treat personality disorders. The most notable exceptions to the usual "50% rule" involve the capacity for social closeness or intimacy (Livesley et al. 1993; Tellegen et al. 1988), for which there is only a moderate (20%) heritability. Some studies (L. A. Baker et al. 1992) indicate that negative emotions are more heritable than positive emotions; this suggests that whereas a difficult temperament can cause unhappiness, happiness depends on having had good experiences. However, the issue remains controversial, since Lykken and Tellegen (1996) have recently reported that genetic factors account for about half of the individual variance on measures of well-being.

Few studies of personality traits have made use of adoption methods. The main exception is the Minnesota study of twins raised apart (Bouchard et al. 1990). The design of this study, comparing personality traits in monozygotic (MZ) and dizygotic (DZ) twins raised together and apart, combines the advantages of twin and adoption studies. The results (Tellegen et al. 1988) have provided strong confirmation for the conclusion that personality is inherited.

The mechanisms by which genetic factors influence personality are complex (Plomin et al. 1997). A given personality trait will not usually be expressed unless several of the genes controlling for that trait are present. Although there have been recent reports of gene associations to major personality dimensions (e.g., Benjamin et al. 1996; Ebstein et al. 1996; Lesch et al. 1996), they all seem to identify only one of several gene loci related to behaviorally measurable traits. Polygenic mechanisms also help to explain why differences between MZ and DZ twins can reflect genetic factors, even when traits themselves do not run strongly in families (Lykken et al. 1992).

Three additional lines of evidence support the biological nature of personality traits. First, some personality traits are associated with biological markers (Cloninger 1987; Eysenck 1991), there being a particularly strong relationship between impulsivity and brain serotonergic activity (Coccaro et al. 1989). Second, the broad dimensions of personality are valid in many different cultures (Eysenck 1991). Third, extreme temperamental characteristics in childhood have an influence on the development of personality (Rothbart and Ahadi 1994). Thus, children with increased fearfulness and irritability may become more neurotic, children with higher activity levels and positive affectivity tend to become more extraverted, children with attentional persistence often become more conscientious, and children who are easily prone to distress tend to have difficulties with attachment.

The environmental factors shaping personality traits are best understood through social learning theory (Bandura 1977). This model hypothesizes that parents influence their children's personality through two mechanisms:

1. Direct reinforcement of behaviors by the parents
2. The child's imitation of observed parental behaviors

This model applies to influences not only from parents but also from other important reinforcers and models in the community.

There is no doubt that parental practices have an important impact on children's behavior. However, as most parents learn from their own experience, there are limits to this influence. Children have their own personalities and are not clay to be shaped by parents. Siblings living in the same family resemble each other little more than if they came from different families (Dunn and Plomin 1990). This is probably why parents with more than one child usually believe in genetics!

One of the surprising findings of twin research concerns the source of environmental influences on personality. For most of the traits reviewed in this book, environmental factors influencing expression are largely "unshared"—that is, not related to living in the same family (Plomin 1994a). As discussed in Chapters 2 and 3, these unshared environmental effects could have a number of possible explanations: 1) siblings receive differential treatment from parents or assume different niches in the family; 2) individuals with different personality traits perceive the same environment differently; and 3) social and community factors outside the family influence personality. All of these mechanisms could be operative, and they have not yet been disentangled.

Some of the residual variance in personality traits reflects the interactions between genes and environment. Children influence the quality of their own environment by shaping the responses of others in accordance with their own traits (Scarr and McCartney 1983). On the positive side, intelligent children seek out a stimulating environment. On the negative side, temperamental abnormalities in children are amplified by the difficulties they create for their parents and peers (Rutter 1987b). This mechanism explains why temperamentally irritable and impulsive children are more likely than those without these traits to experience abuse and neglect in their families (Rutter and Quinton 1984).

The effects of temperament on personality act to "bend the twig"—that is, to set limits on what characteristics can eventually predominate in an individual. Since environmental factors account for more than half of the variance in traits (Livesley et al. 1993), these factors will determine the final shape of personality. The discontinuities between infantile temperament and later personality (Chess and Thomas 1990) reflect the crucial role for environmental factors in development. Interactions between parenting and temperament (i.e., "goodness of fit") best explain these findings.

Personality Traits and Personality Disorders

Personality disorders are pathological exaggerations of normal traits (Paris 1993, 1996a). The relation between traits and disorders therefore involves a process of *amplification*. If this view is correct, there should be no sharp break between normal personality and pathological personality. Traits would become disorders only at some cutoff point at which they result in significant dysfunction.

This concept of continuity between traits and disorders has been fairly well supported by empirical research. For example, in large-scale studies of twins in the community and of patients in psychiatric clinics, Livesley et al. (1993) failed to find any sharp cutoff between normal and pathological personality dimensions.

By and large, a wide range of variability in personality is compatible with normality. There is room in the world for both extraverts and introverts, for both those who worry and those who do not, for both those who are emotional and those who are not, and for both those who are cautious and those more likely to jump into things.

Any set of behaviors can be adaptive when applied in appropriate circumstances yet maladaptive when applied in inappropriate circumstances. Thus, extraverts tend to thrive in a setting that requires sociability, but they have difficulty when they do not receive social reinforcements. Introverts are productive in settings that require the capacity to work alone, but often they are in danger of becoming isolated. People who worry are more likely to see trouble before it hits them, but they can also anticipate troubles that are unlikely to occur. People who do not worry can have a better life, but this works only as long as all goes well. People who are highly emotional can feel more joyous and alive. Yet, people who are unemotional are better able to tolerate hard times. People who are cautious make fewer mistakes. Yet, people who are impulsive fare better when a rapid response is required.

Personality traits are alternative evolutionary strategies, each of which is more or less adaptive depending on environmental demands (Beck and Freeman 1990). It is when these traits are discordant with social expectations that psychopathology ensues. Traits that do not meet social demands will significantly interfere with functioning. Moreover, when traits are expressed rigidly and maladaptively, they can cause even more dysfunction.

Eventually, when traits are amplified to the point that they lead to social dysfunction, the clinical picture can come to meet the criteria for the general definition of a personality disorder in DSM-IV (American Psychiatric Association 1994). These criteria describe enduring patterns of inner experience and behavior that deviate from cultural expectations, that are inflexible and pervasive, that lead to clinically significant distress or impairment, and that are stable over time.

DSM divides the personality disorders into 10 categories, grouped into three clusters:

- Cluster A: schizoid, paranoid, and schizotypal
- Cluster B: antisocial, narcissistic, borderline, and histrionic
- Cluster C: avoidant, dependent, and compulsive

It cannot be too strongly emphasized that this classification scheme is, at best, provisional. It is likely that new methods of categorization, based on a better understanding of trait dimensions, will eventually be developed. At present, the three clusters might have more overall validity than any of the individual 10 categories. There is a great deal of overlap among individual disorders, with each diagnosable disorder usually accompanied by at least one additional Axis II diagnosis (Pfohl et al. 1986). Most of the comorbidity occurs within clusters.

For example, in Cluster B, each specific category of diagnosis depends on the patient's gender and symptom severity (Paris 1997). Thus, severe levels of impulsivity might lead to a diagnosis of antisocial personality disorder in men or of borderline personality disorder in women, while less severe problems, perhaps centering on instability in relationships, might lead to a diagnosis of narcissistic personality disorder in men or of histrionic personality disorder in women. Similar considerations apply to the overlap of disorders in Clusters A and C (Paris 1996a).

Whatever the validity of the categories, the process by which traits develop into disorders requires a theoretical model. We need a mechanism to explain 1) the amplification of traits to disorders and 2) the specificity of disorders.

In understanding the amplification process, it is important to bear in mind that no one etiological factor is a sufficient cause of personality pathology. Biological, psychological, and social factors are all involved, so that the process depends on multiple risk factors. These risks are buffered by protective factors that make the amplification of traits less likely.

The type of personality disorder that develops depends on individual differences in trait profiles. For example, excessive impulsivity and emotionality may increase the risk for a Cluster B disorder, while excessive introversion and worry can increase the risk for a Cluster C disorder.

Some personality disorder researchers believe that since traits and disorders lie on a continuum, dimensional measures provide a better way of classifying personality pathology. Eysenck (1991), Costa and Widiger (1994), and Cloninger (1987) have all suggested ways in which the dimensions in their respective schemata could be used to reconstruct the disorders defined in DSM. However, given the overlapping nature of individual disorders, it might be more useful to relate trait dimensions to the Axis II clusters. Based on phenomenology, Table 3 suggests relationships between the clusters and these broad dimensional schemata.

▨ Biological Predispositions to Personality Disorders

The predisposing biological factors in personality disorders are largely unknown (Nigg and Goldsmith 1994). We have more theories than solid evidence. However, only a biological model can account for the fact that individuals with all the psychosocial risk factors for personality disorders do not necessarily develop these disorders, and that the same risks produce different personality disorders in different people.

Theoretically, one set of predisposing factors might be unusually intense traits or combinations of traits. Such traits, particularly if amplified, would be more likely to produce discordance with social expectations.

TABLE 3. Hypothesized relationships between personality dimensions and the Axis I clusters of personality disorders

Hypothesis	Cluster A	Cluster B	Cluster C
Eysenck (1991)[1]	↓E, ↑P	↑N, ↑E, ↑P	↑N, ↓E
Five Factor (Costa and McRae 1988)[2]	↓E, ↓A	↑N, ↓C, ↑O, ±↓A	↓E, ↑N, ±↑A
Cloninger (1987)[3]	↓NS, ↑HA, ↓RD	↑NS, ↓HA, ±↓RD	↓NS, ↑HA, ±↑RD

[1]N = neuroticism; E = extraversion; P = psychoticism.
[2]N = neuroticism; E = extraversion; O = openness to experience; A = agreeableness; C = conscientiousness.
[3]NS = novelty seeking; HA = harm avoidance; RD = reward dependence.

Siever and Davis (1991) have developed a model based on this principle. Individuals with personality disorders would begin life with an unusually high intensity of one or several temperamental characteristics. The abnormalities would appear on one or more of four dimensions: emotional instability, impulsivity, social anxiety, or cognitive instability. Those predisposed to develop personality disorders might lack other, more adaptive traits that could mediate these temperamental vulnerabilities.

The schema proposed by Cloninger et al. (1993) makes similar predictions. Thus, individuals with high novelty seeking and low harm avoidance will be impulsive, which will place them at risk for personality disorders that lie in the B cluster. However, high persistence would buffer the effects of high impulsivity, making personality pathology less likely.

Both of these theories are heuristic but require a great deal more data. Evidence for biological factors in the personality disorders will require three lines of research: 1) estimates of heritability derived from twin and adoption studies; 2) studies of biological markers; and 3) prospective studies of temperamentally difficult children.

The first line of research, measuring heritability in the personality disorders, has thus far yielded limited information. Most studies have measured traits by examining overt behaviors rather than by determining formal diagnoses. For example, adoption studies show that traits of criminality have a moderate degree of heritability (Cloninger et al. 1982; Crowe 1974; Mednick et al. 1984). Yet we do not know how well these findings apply to diagnosable cases of antisocial personality disorder.

Many twin studies of personality disorders have been carried out by the Norwegian psychologist Sven Torgersen. In all his studies, Torgersen (1980, 1983, 1984, 1991; Torgersen et al. 1993) found that when traits and disorders were measured in the same patients, differences in MZ versus DZ concordance were much greater for either traits or symptoms than for disorders. In the Cluster B disorders, impulsivity, rather than borderline personality, was heritable (Torgersen 1991). In the Cluster C disorders, social anxiety, rather than avoidant or dependent personality, had a stronger genetic loading (Torgersen 1983). Similarly, obsessiveness, rather than compulsive personality disorder, was heritable (Torgersen 1980, 1991).

Torgersen's findings have generally been confirmed by other researchers. For example, Kendler et al. (1981, 1984), examining Cluster A disorders, found genetic factors to be more strongly related to certain symptoms, such as thought disorder, than to the diagnosis of schizotypal personality.

However, this does not mean that personality disorders are not heritable. As pointed out by Nigg and Goldsmith (1994), genetic factors could play a substantial role in determining *extreme* levels on the continuum of personality traits. Moreover, if, as shown by Livesley et al. (1993), there are genetic loadings in the traits underlying these diagnoses, personality disorders should be at least partially heritable.

Recently, Torgersen (1996) conducted a study that showed, for the first time, that many of the DSM-IV personality disorders have a significant degree of heritability. Collecting 235 twin pairs from around Norway in which at least one proband had a diagnosable personality disorder, he found that several of the personality disorders have a major genetic component. The results are more generalizable for those disorders that had a high frequency in the sample: borderline personality disorder (34 pairs) and avoidant personality disorder (28 pairs). The findings demonstrated a high genetic loading (over 50% of the variance) for both of these categories, as well as for two others: narcissistic and compulsive personality disorders.

A second method of examining genetic factors in the personality disorders involves looking for biological markers. Again, the results indicate that traits are much more closely related to biological factors than are disorders (Siever and Davis 1991). Thus far, there have been no specific markers associated with the diagnoses in DSM-IV (Paris 1996a). When biological markers *have* been identified in personality disorder patients, they have been more strongly related either to comorbid diagnoses on Axis I or to underlying traits (McGuffin and Thapar 1992; Nigg and Goldsmith 1994).

For example, patients with impulsive personality disorders had abnormal dexamethasone suppression and decreased rapid eye movement (REM) latency only when they were also depressed (Gunderson and Phillips 1991). In another example, male patients with Cluster B diagnoses had a decreased response to fenfluramine challenge (measuring decreased activity in the serotonergic system) that was strongly related to traits of impulsive aggression but only weakly related to specific diagnostic categories such as antisocial or borderline personality disorder (Coccaro et al. 1989). Most recently, low levels of serotonin metabolites in newborns have been associated with a family history of antisocial personality disorder (Constantino 1997).

Future advances in biotechnology will no doubt identify other biological markers. However, as in the past, most markers will probably continue to be more strongly associated with traits than disorders. As discussed earlier, trait profiles do not predict whether individuals will develop a personality disorder, but instead determine the specific *category* of disorder to which individuals are vulnerable (Paris 1996a).

Thus far, the evidence remains insufficient to provide definitive support for Siever's hypothesis that unusually intense levels of traits increase the risk for personality disorders. However, if these predispositions are indeed necessary conditions for personality disorders, we need more precise ways to identify them, probably methods using biological markers and gene linkages.

A third line of research involves longitudinal studies of children. The fact that personality disorders begin early in life and demonstrate chronicity over time could be a reflection of their origins in temperament.

There are demonstrable long-term effects in adult life of a "difficult" temperament during infancy (e.g., Chess and Thomas 1990). Temperamentally difficult children have an overall increased risk for adult psychopathology, although we do not know whether personality disorders are one of the outcomes. Prospective studies following children with extreme temperaments (Kagan 1994; Maziade et al. 1990) will help to answer these questions. Since these cohorts are only now reaching adolescence, we will have to wait a few more years to know whether they show personality pathology as adults.

The temperamental precursors of personality disorders are probably different in each Axis II cluster. Disorders in Cluster A often run in the same families as schizophrenia (see Chapter 8). In the B cluster, relatives tend to share traits associated with impulsive or affective personality dimensions (Silverman et al. 1991). Antisocial personality begins with conduct disorder in childhood, but we do not know the extent to which conduct symptoms reflect a temperamental component (see Chapter 14). Moreover, conduct disorder is a common precursor of personality disorders in all three clusters (Bernstein et al. 1996).

Kagan's (1994) work is of particular relevance for the disorders in the C cluster. Temperamental variability, in the form of extreme shyness beginning in infancy ("behavioral inhibition"), can be associated either with anxiety disorders (see Chapter 10) or with avoidant or dependent personality disorders (Paris 1998). This trait is also protective against the development of delinquency. In Kagan's cohort, anxious personality traits remained stable in a large percentage of cases up to early adolescence, with only about one-third of these children overcoming their shyness. Behavioral inhibition was more likely to persist over time if parents responded to this trait with overprotection rather than by encouraging their children to overcome shyness (Kagan 1994). This observation confirms the view of Chess and Thomas (1990) that temperamental difficulties are most persistent when there is a lack of "goodness of fit" between children and parents.

In summary, temperamental factors do not by themselves determine whether individuals will develop personality disorders. However, certain temperamental profiles are associated with an increased likelihood of being exposed to environmental risks: impulsive children are more likely to enter into conflict with their parents, and anxious children are more likely to be overprotected. These stressors may be the crucial determinants of the pathways between traits and disorders.

Psychological Stressors in the Personality Disorders

A large body of research (see summary in Paris 1996a) shows that patients with personality disorders report an unusually large number of negative childhood experiences. These reports describe adversities such as early separation from or loss of parents, abnormalities in parenting, emotional neglect, and traumatic experiences. The common factor seems to be family dysfunction.

However, all of the findings from research on the psychological factors in the personality disorders depend on the validity of retrospective reports of childhood experiences. In view of the vagaries of long-term memory (see Chapter 11) and the tendency for perceptions of the past to be filtered through the present (Parker 1992), we must view this evidence with caution. Retrospective reports can sometimes be validated (Maughan and Rutter 1997) but they cannot consistently be trusted.

It is entirely possible that the findings summarized above only reflect how dysfunctional adults account for their present difficulties, i.e., by blaming their families. Moreover, the tendency to blame one's parents for life problems can be reinforced by psychotherapists as well as by the prevailing climate of opinion transmitted through the media (see discussion in Ofshe and Watters 1994). In addition, all measures of childhood experiences have a heritable component (Plomin and Bergeman 1991), reflecting the fact that perceptions of life events are, at least in part, a reflection of personality traits (see Chapter 3).

Early separation from or loss of parents is the most objective of all risk factors, and therefore creates fewer problems through distortion of memory, or through the processing of experience by personality. Even so, the long-term effects of losing a parent depend on many factors other than the simple facts of death or divorce (Tennant 1988).

Early losses are rather common in patients with personality disorders. In a large sample of both males and females with various Axis II diagnoses studied by the author and his colleagues, about half had lost a parent, either through divorce or death, before age 16, and a quarter before age 5 (Paris et al. 1994a, 1994b). (This rate is genuinely high, since the subjects in this sample had grown up prior to the recent "epidemic" of divorce.)

The empirical evidence suggests that parental divorce is a *relative* risk factor for long-term problems in children (Hetherington et al.

1985; Rutter and Maughan 1997; J. Wallerstein 1989). Other things being equal, it is better to be brought up in an intact family. The obvious exceptions involve mental illness in a parent or family violence, in which case separation can even be positive for children (Rutter 1989). However, family breakdown does not, *by itself,* create a long-term risk for psychopathology. The reason is that the effects of separation from or loss of a parent during childhood depend on their interactions with other risk factors (Rutter 1989; Tennant 1988). On the whole, a pathological outcome is most likely when one negative experience leads to another, producing a "cascade" effect.

Studies of community populations of children of divorce are therefore reassuring (Hetherington et al. 1985). As with other adversities, resilience is the rule. The problem is that although divorce does not *necessarily* cause a cascade, it often does. Moreover, family breakdown may have a different effect, not seen in normal populations, in children who are temperamentally vulnerable.

Abnormal parenting during childhood is another risk factor for developing personality disorders in adulthood. Many studies have shown that patients with personality pathology are more likely to have had parents with psychiatric disorders. For example, the strongest risk factor for antisocial personality is criminality or antisocial behavior in a parent (L. N. Robins 1966). Individuals with borderline personality disorder are more likely to have had parents with personality disorders, chronic depression, or substance abuse (Links et al. 1988b).

Although these associations could reflect common genetic vulnerabilities, it seems commonsensical to assume that living with a mentally ill parent is a stressor in its own right. There might even be a particular risk for children if a parent has a personality disorder, since, unlike intermittent symptomatic disorders, personality pathology has a *continuous* effect on parenting capacity.

Additional evidence for the negative effects of having a parent with a personality disorder comes from research in children. In our own center (M. Weiss et al. 1996), we examined a high-risk sample of latency-aged children (i.e., age 5 years to puberty) of mothers with personality disorders. Over half of these children had features of conduct disorder or oppositional defiant disorder, either of which can be a precursor of adult personality disorders.

Abnormal parenting can also be measured through the quality of parent–child relationships. Clinicians (e.g., G. Adler 1985) have suggested that personality disorders can be a result of emotional neglect during childhood. This possibility can be investigated empirically by retrospective measures of the quality of parenting.

The best-known self-report instrument for this purpose is the Parental Bonding Index (Parker 1983). This scale derives its constructs from theories of child development, which define the tasks of parenting in terms of two basic dimensions: providing affection and allowing autonomy (Rowe 1981). Research using this measure (e.g., Paris et al. 1994a, 1994b) shows that personality disorder patients report serious problems in bonding with their parents, including both a lack of affection (neglect) and a lack of autonomy (overcontrol). However, problems in parental bonding are not very specific to any category of disorder, or even to the personality disorders as a group; such problems are also reported by patients with many other psychiatric diagnoses (Parker 1983).

Another way of determining the quality of parenting involves self-report measures of family structure. The best known of these instruments is the Family Environment Scale (FES; Moos and Moos 1986). FES subscales describe a family's cohesion and organization, its emotional expressiveness, and its encouragement of independence. Studies using the FES have found differences between personality disorder categories; for example, patients with borderline personality disorder tend to have low family cohesion (Feldman et al. 1995; Ogata et al. 1990b), while the families of patients with dependent personality disorder are characterized by low emotional expression and overcontrol (Head et al. 1991). Again, these findings may only reflect personality traits shared by parents and children. However, they could also be interpreted as suggesting an etiological relationship between specific types of family experience and specific categories of personality disorders.

In converging evidence from many studies, personality disorder patients commonly report traumatic events, particularly childhood sexual abuse and/or childhood physical abuse (see reviews in Paris 1994, 1996a). These reports are particularly frequent among patients with borderline personality disorder (Herman et al. 1989; Links et al. 1988a; Ogata et al. 1990a; Paris et al. 1994a, 1994b). Cross-sectional studies of "borderline" children (Guzder et al. 1996), some of whom may have early forms of personality disorder, show very similar risk factors and avoid the problem of retrospective distortion.

The problem is that there is little specificity in the relationship between trauma and borderline personality disorder, and even less between trauma and the personality disorders as a whole (Paris 1994). Therefore, even when we find a high frequency of child abuse in borderline patients, such abuse is only one of several risk factors for the disorder. These findings cannot pinpoint any precise causal pathways to borderline personality.

We need to place the relationships between trauma and personality disorders within the context of community studies of child abuse (Browne and Finkelhor 1986; Fergusson et al. 1996a, 1996b; Malinovsky-Rummell and Hansen 1993). As reviewed in Chapter 11, even though child abuse is a risk factor for a wide range of psychological symptoms in adulthood, about 80% of adults with abuse histories show no demonstrable psychopathology. These community studies also show that the long-term sequelae of abuse experiences depend on the severity of trauma. However, most reported child abuse is of *low* severity. Patients with personality disorders are not different from community populations, in that most reports of sexual abuse involve low-severity events: usually *single* incidents associated with perpetrators who are *not* family members (Paris et al. 1994a, 1994b).

In summary, although child abuse can be associated with pathological sequelae, the presence of abuse histories in patients fails to provide an adequate explanation of their current symptomatology. The effects of trauma can be fully understood only through their interactions with other risk factors and with biological predispositions.

Moreover, as discussed in Chapter 11, there are no clinical symptoms that can be used as "markers" for trauma. Some researchers (e.g., Herman and van der Kolk 1987) have claimed that dissociation is such a marker. However, in community studies of dissociation (Tillman et al. 1994; Irwin 1996; Mulder et al. 1998; Nash et al. 1993), when intercorrelated risk factors, such as emotional neglect in the family, are taken into account, there are no specific relationships between dissociation and child abuse. Our research group (Zweig-Frank et al. 1994a, 1994b, 1994c, 1994d) came to similar conclusions about dissociative phenomena in borderline personality disorder; such phenomena are more a reflection of the disorder than of any particular life history.

In conclusion, the effects of *any* of the psychological stressors that are risk factors for personality disorders can be better understood in the context of interactions with biological predispositions. A number of lines of evidence support this way of looking at the evidence.

First, the association of negative events with personality disorders is partly due to common traits leading to pathological behavior in care-takers. Since the first-degree relatives of personality disorder patients themselves have impulsive or affectively unstable personality traits (Silverman et al. 1991), traumatized children are likely to have parents with similar characteristics. Not even separation from or loss of parents is a random environmental event, since it can be driven by personality traits in parents that make family breakdown more likely (Rutter 1987a). Similarly, both diagnosable parental psychopathology and parental neglect may derive from dysfunctional personality traits that reflect a genetic vulnerability shared by children and parents.

Second, temperamentally difficult children are significantly more likely to be mistreated in their families (Rutter and Quinton 1984). An irritable child is much more likely to be abused, and much less likely to be treated well. Alternatively, parents can respond overprotectively to a child with a difficult temperament, failing to provide the limits and boundaries that are known to help contain impulsivity and affective instability.

Third, the effects of negative events in childhood are mediated by individual differences in cognitive schemata (Finkelhor 1988). Some people have traits, such as neuroticism, that make them more vulnerable to negative events. Other, more resilient people react less strongly to life's vicissitudes and are less susceptible to adverse events. Any theory of the etiology of the personality disorders needs to account for why different children perceive the same environment differently.

In summary, traumatic experiences, however distressing, have greater impact on those who are constitutionally predisposed to personality pathology. Interactions between predispositions and stressors are crucial to understanding the psychological factors in the personality disorders.

Social Factors in the Personality Disorders

The basic dimensions of personality are similar all over the world (Eysenck 1982). However, there are also cross-cultural differences, usually of the magnitude of about half a standard deviation (Eysenck 1982). This shows that societies can, at least to some extent, shape personality traits. Social expectations encourage some kinds of behavior and suppress others.

Societies differ in their ability to tolerate different traits. Thus, traditional societies are more tolerant of dependence, and most individuals are expected to conform to group and family norms. On the other hand, modern societies expect high levels of autonomy, and most individuals are expected to develop their own career paths and to find their own spouses and friends (Paris 1996a). These expectations are highly stressful for those who cannot easily meet them.

Personality disorders, as defined by Axis II of DSM, can be diagnosed in clinical populations all over the world (Loranger et al. 1994). However, if societies shape personality, then disorders should have a differential prevalence across cultures. This hypothesis is ripe for investigation.

Thus far, the most solid evidence for cultural shaping of personality relates to antisocial personality disorder. This condition, which has shown a high and dramatically increasing prevalence in North America (L. N. Robins and Regier 1991), has a surprisingly low prevalence in certain East Asian societies, such as Taiwan (Hwu et al. 1989). The most likely explanation is that North American families are much more likely to produce the risk factors for this condition, such as failure to discipline children effectively (L. N. Robins 1966). In contrast, the traditional structure of Taiwanese families and society creates a strong atmosphere of discipline and suppresses most of the impulsive behaviors in children that characterize conduct disorder.

In accordance with the observation that the most important environmental influences on personality are "unshared," the social factors influencing the personality disorders may depend in part on the availability of attachment figures outside the nuclear family and on access to social networks. However, as discussed in Chapter 3, children vary in their constitutional capacity to make use of these networks.

Social factors can be used to define an overall measure of health in the community, which Leighton et al. (1963) have called *social integration*. In contrast, *social disintegration* is characterized by a breakdown of extended family ties, a loss of social networks, a lack of community ties, a normlessness related to the loss of consensual values, and difficulties in developing and maintaining social roles. These social conditions may constitute risk factors for personality disorders (Paris 1996a).

A Predisposition–Stress Model of the Personality Disorders

The psychosocial factors influencing the personality disorders are all associated with *statistical* risks rather than with strongly predictable effects. The relative weakness of these associations makes sense if psychosocial risks are likely to be pathogenic only in interaction with a genetic vulnerability. These observations provide support for a model in which personality disorders are the outcome of interactions between predispositions (traits) and stressors (psychosocial risk factors).

A predisposition–stress model of this kind was first suggested by M. H. Stone (1980) for borderline personality disorder. Similar ideas have more recently been elaborated by Linehan (1993) and Paris (1994) in their books on borderline personality disorder. Parallel models have been proposed for all of the personality disorders by Beck and Freeman (1990), M. H. Stone (1993), and Paris (1996a).

Let us examine how we might combine the effects of biological, psychological, and social factors into a predisposition–stress model. The biological variability in personality traits reflects temperament. However, a wide range of trait variability is compatible with normality, and trait variations are insufficient by themselves to account for the amplification of traits into disorders. On the other hand, traits are the main determinant of which type of personality disorder can develop. Thus, disorders characterized by extraversion, such as those in the impulsive cluster, cannot appear in those who are introverted. Conversely, disorders characterized by introversion, such as those in the odd and anxious clusters, cannot emerge in those who are extraverted.

Every individual has a mixture of traits: some more adaptive, others less adaptive. An unusual intensity of certain traits may lower the threshold at which stressors can trigger a personality disorder. The best example of this pathway concerns the emotional instability and impulsivity that, particularly in combination, are associated with borderline personality disorder.

Psychological and social factors are the crucial determinants of whether underlying traits lead to overt disorders. However, these factors do not by themselves cause personality disorders. This conclusion is supported by the evidence that most children are resilient, even in the face of the most severe stressors, ranging from socioeconomic deprivation to severe parental pathology. Without temperamental vulnerability, children usually have sufficient resilience to compensate for most adversities.

Personality disorders, therefore, are prime examples of gene–environment interactions. Some of the traits underlying personality disorders increase both *exposure* and *susceptibility* to environmental factors (see Chapter 3). Both impulsivity alone (associated with antisocial personality disorder) and the combination of impulsivity and affective instability (associated with borderline personality disorder) are temperamental factors that make it more likely that children will be either badly treated or mishandled. Moreover, temperamental factors, such as high neuroticism, can make children more susceptible to stressors. These interactions between temperament and environment could play a crucial role in the pathways to impulsive disorders.

Similarly, an anxious temperament leads to social anxiety and avoidance, characteristics that interfere with peer relationships and that can make children even more anxious and withdrawn. Moreover, anxious children are difficult to raise and tend to elicit either overprotection or rejection from parents. Thus, genetic factors influence both exposure and susceptibility to environmental stressors.

For most patients, the risk of developing personality pathology is greatly increased by stressful life experiences. Although acute stressors need not necessarily distort personality structure (Lazarus and Folkman 1984), chronic adversities are more likely to have an amplifying effect on traits. Yet, psychological protective factors, consisting of positive life experiences, can buffer these risk factors. Stressful experiences inside the family can also be buffered by extrafamilial attachments, which have been consistently shown to protect children at risk.

The role of social factors in this model would be to influence the threshold at which traits become amplified into disorders. Social factors can be protective, as when strong community supports buffer biological and psychological risks. Alternatively, social factors can be risks in their own right, as in the case of sociocultural disintegration.

The etiological pathways to personality disorders will be different for different diagnostic categories. Disorders in Cluster A lie in the schizophrenic spectrum and are highly heritable. Cluster B disorders derive from interactions between impulsive or affective traits and family dysfunction. Cluster C disorders derive from the amplification of anxious traits by psychosocial stressors.

Summary

Many unanswered questions remain about the etiology of the personality disorders. We will need a great deal more research before we can begin to understand how these disorders develop. Most particularly, there is a lack of longitudinal studies of children followed into adulthood, which could define more precisely which risk factors are most etiologically crucial.

Research on the personality disorders also offers a better perspective on the validity of the doctrine of the primacy of early experience (see Chapter 3). Since personality disorders begin early in life and are difficult to treat, it has often been assumed that the most important stressors that lead to their development derive from childhood. However, as we have seen in this chapter, it is more likely that the early onset and chronicity of these disorders are a reflection of their origins in temperament.

Thus, the personality disorders, far from demonstrating how childhood experiences are the crucial factors in the development of adult psychopathology, provide one of the best exemplars of the interactions between nature and nurture.

PART III

Implications

16

Clinical Implications

Mental health clinicians have the task of changing their patients' minds. In recent years, it has become increasingly attractive to produce this change through neurochemical means. Compared with psychopharmacological agents used in the past, modern psychiatric drugs are more effective, have a wider spectrum of efficacy, and cause fewer side effects.

The trend toward a biological orientation in psychiatry has become so pervasive that, for some practitioners, clinical work has come to consist of little but brief checkups and the writing of prescriptions. In many settings, nonmedical mental health workers have become the primary caregivers, with most psychotherapy being provided by nonpsychiatrists, while family doctors are becoming more and more adept in psychopharmacology. The discipline of psychiatry is struggling to define the ways in which it remains unique.

Applying a broader model of the causes of psychopathology could help develop an alternative to this fragmentation of mental health care. Psychiatry is unique in crossing the boundaries between many disciplines. Its clinical practitioners therefore need to be *eclectic*. They also need to be committed to *evidence-based* practice, offering patients treatments that have been demonstrated to be effective in empirical research.

This chapter will aim to show how a predisposition–stress model of psychopathology can guide clinical work. In it I will suggest two directions for the future: eclecticism and evidence-based practice. To understand why clinical practice must be integrative, we will examine the problems associated with reductionism, both biological and environmental. Two of the most common clinical problems in psychiatry—the treatment of major depressive disorder and the psychotherapy of personality disorders—will be used to illustrate these principles.

The point of view taken in this chapter is hardly unique and has been developed by many other writers (e.g., Eisenberg 1995). Most recently, Gabbard and Goodwin (1996), who are, respectively, a well-known psychoanalyst and a leading researcher in biological psychiatry, have written eloquently about the value of using a stress–diathesis model to understand mental disorders. Such a model allows practitioners to offer patients a broader set of treatment options.

Biological Reductionism in Psychiatry

In principle, psychiatrists are committed to holism. Yet, some of the most serious mistakes made in the past were based on misguided attempts to consider "the whole patient." By trying to take into account the complexity of the individual, practitioners lost sight of their responsibility to relieve distress. Today, by reducing complex syndromes to target symptoms that can respond to specific drugs, we can often treat patients more effectively. Reductionism also has its good points!

The author of this book is old enough to have visited mental hospitals before the introduction of neuroleptics. As an undergraduate student in psychology, I observed the grim fates of patients in these institutions. Later on, first as a medical student and then as a resident, I was expected to manage a wide variety of outpatients by exploring their personal histories, without being taught any practical means to provide relief for their symptoms. Clinicians today have the benefit of many more options.

Over the last few decades, there has been an exponential increase in knowledge of the neurosciences. This "biological revolution" has dramatically changed psychiatry. The study of neurotransmitter activity is at the cutting edge of contemporary theory and research and is the conceptual basis for developing even better forms of pharmacological treatment. The clinical implications of advances in psychiatric genetics have also been enormous. In the foreseeable future, by studying our patients' genomes, we will be able to inform them about their vulnerabilities to mental disorders.

These felicitous developments have also been associated with some negative trends. There are clinicians for whom history-taking consists of little more than a checklist used to determine whether the patient meets criteria for a DSM diagnosis. Therapy may then consist only of prescribing drugs appropriate for that category. Unfortunately, this picture is not a caricature!

Errors in practice are often based on misunderstandings in theory. Reductionistic models of psychopathology lead to reductionistic methods of treatment. Clinicians may forget that psychiatric diagnoses are rarely homogeneous entities. As I have argued in this book, most forms of psychopathology lie on a spectrum in which overt disorders emerge from complex interactions between predispositions and stressors. Moreover, similar clinical symptoms can arise from very different pathways. In some cases, strong predispositions will be operating, while in others, the influence of the environment will be the determining factor. Clinical observations cannot usually separate these cases.

Patients with the same diagnosis can be very different; therefore, no simple algorithm determines the right choice of treatment. Throughout this book, I have emphasized the importance of *individual differences*. The art of medicine also involves *individualizing* therapy. Good clinical practice means taking the uniqueness of every patient into account. The treatment of major depression is an example demonstrating this principle.

◼ Beyond Reductionism: The Treatment of Major Depression

The biological revolution in psychiatry has profoundly affected the treatment of major depressive disorder. It has become almost standard practice to prescribe an antidepressant for patients who meet the DSM criteria for this diagnosis. If patients do not respond to the first drug prescribed, they are labeled "treatment resistant" and are offered a more complex pharmacological regimen.

Biological reductionism runs the danger of reducing patient autonomy. Some people suffering from depression may be comforted by the belief that their distress is entirely attributable to "chemical imbalances." Other patients use biology as an excuse to avoid dealing with life problems that must be addressed to reduce the risk of relapse.

Depressed patients are very heterogeneous (see Chapter 9). The most severe cases of depression, associated either with a bipolar illness or with psychotic or melancholic symptoms, have the strongest genetic predispositions. Patients with less severe depressions carry a weaker genetic load, and their illness is more influenced by environmental precipitants. It is therefore logical to provide different treatment options for different forms of illness.

Moreover, the criteria for a diagnosis of major depressive disorder are very broad. Patients can meet them even when they are sleeping normally, maintaining a good appetite, and not considering suicide. To meet the diagnostic criteria in DSM, it is sufficient to feel depressed most of the time, to have lost interest in daily activities, to feel excessively tired, to have difficulty concentrating, and to dislike oneself. However, it is far from clear that all patients meeting these criteria suffer from the same illness.

Moreover, the assumption that a diagnosis of major depression, by itself, provides sufficient information to make intelligent decisions about the treatment of depression is not supported by empirical research.

In fact, DSM-IV (American Psychiatric Association 1994) does not define any of its categories on the basis of treatment response. With the exception of the psychoses, there is little evidence that Axis I diagnoses predict the effectiveness of *any* specific form of treatment.

Research does not support the idea that every patient with major depression *must* be treated with drugs. The National Institute of Mental Health (NIMH) Collaborative Study of Depression (Elkin et al. 1989) found that for most patients, several different forms of psychotherapy yielded results equivalent to those obtained with antidepressants. (Positive results were, however, somewhat slower to emerge.) Only in severe cases (i.e., those with melancholia) were antidepressants clearly superior to psychotherapy. Thus, when the criteria for melancholia are absent, there is little justification for prescribing antidepressants *routinely*. Psychotherapy alone can be a perfectly adequate treatment.

Patient preferences play a crucial role in these clinical decisions. Some patients are only interested in receiving pharmacotherapy for their symptoms. We can usually accept these preferences, given that antidepressant therapy yields positive results in a wide range of patients, including many with milder depressions, and in about half of patients with dysthymia (Kocsis et al. 1991). However, in doing so, we need not think of antidepressants as correcting "chemical imbalances." Rather, these agents probably act to break vicious circles, allowing patients to escape from negative-feedback loops between depressed affect and depression-driven behaviors.

Some depressed patients dislike taking pills, insisting that they "only want to talk." In most cases, unless the depression is severe, clinicians can feel secure that psychotherapy will be effective. Even in melancholic depression, patients sometimes get better without drugs. This is probably because the process of therapy, by its very nature, has a striking effect on morale (J. Frank and J. B. Frank 1991).

Many patients with depression will prefer to receive both pharmacological and psychotherapeutic therapy. Combined treatment has the advantage of providing faster symptomatic relief while addressing the factors that lead to chronicity. Klerman et al. (1974) have shown that if clinicians prescribe both psychotherapy and drugs to all patients, they "cover all the bases." (This does not mean, however, that everyone needs both forms of treatment.)

Some patients will leave treatment decisions to the therapist. Because patients often improve to a surprising degree as a result of a single contact (Howard et al. 1986), it may be wise to hold off a final decision about whether to treat with drugs or psychotherapy until the second session. If patients with nonmelancholic depression improve between the first and second contacts, we will have saved them a great deal of trouble by waiting before prescribing.

The treatment of depression has to take the danger of chronicity into account. Follow-up studies show that major depression has a high rate of relapse (Shea et al. 1992). Some of this chronicity may be rooted in biological predispositions, which can be strong enough to produce a relapse whenever drug treatment is interrupted. Alternatively, chronicity may be a result of "kindling" (see Chapter 9), so that each episode makes the next one more likely. For these reasons, a certain percentage of depressed patients need long-term pharmacological therapy.

However, *personality* is another important factor influencing the chronicity of depression. Research demonstrates that the presence of *any* Axis II comorbidity makes it much less likely that drug therapy will be successful in managing depressive symptoms (Shea et al. 1990). Moreover, such comorbidity is far from uncommon: diagnosable personality disorders are present in at least a quarter of depressed patients (Patience et al. 1995) and are even more common in early-onset depression (Fava et al. 1996). Finally, the *majority* of patients with dysthymia have significant Axis II comorbidity (Pepper et al. 1995).

These findings have important clinical implications. There is an important subgroup of depressed patients who need other forms of treatment beyond the prescription of drugs. A recent study (Wiborg and Dahl 1996) showed that when brief psychodynamic psychotherapy was added to psychopharmacological management, relapse of panic disorder became much less frequent. It seems likely that similar findings will emerge for major depression. Research on the psychotherapy of depressed patients (Barkham et al. 1997; Kopta et al. 1994) has already shown that although the acute symptoms of mood disorder respond quickly to contact with a therapist, characterological components associated with chronicity require longer interventions.

Many clinicians seem to have forgotten the principle that depression is rooted in personality. This is an insight that has long been a defining construct in psychiatry. It has also earned important empirical support from studies of depressed patients (Coyne and Whiffen 1995). This principles helps us as therapists to see each patient as a person and to take into account important individual differences that go beyond diagnosis.

This is why it is insufficient to label *all* patients who fail to respond to antidepressant drugs as "treatment resistant." Undoubtedly, many patients improve when we switch antidepressants or add mood-stabilizing agents. However, if changing medications is all we do, we may miss other significant factors that maintain depressed mood. By failing to take the time to make a systematic assessment of personality, clinicians reduce their ability to predict which patients are most likely to benefit from symptomatic treatment.

Even in schizophrenia, a disorder known to be strongly biological, drug treatment alone is sufficient only to manage the acute stages of the illness (May 1970). In the long term, rehabilitative psychosocial interventions markedly reduce the risk of relapse (G. W. Brown et al. 1994; Hogarty et al. 1991).

As discussed in Chapter 7, diagnoses in psychiatry are useful modes of communication but should not be thought of as "real" entities. This is why diagnosis provides an overall guideline to understanding patients, but is usually insufficient for making a detailed treatment plan.

It was only when biological psychiatry became the dominant paradigm in psychiatry that more precise diagnostic practices based on specific and well-defined criteria became a practical possibility. To provide a comprehensive assessment of cases, DSM developed a five-axis system. The problem is that clinicians rarely use all the axes! Practitioners have trouble thinking multidimensionally and like to convert complex clinical syndromes into easily understood algorithms.

Once they have made an Axis I diagnosis, many clinicians are satisfied that they have done their job. The main reason for this narrow approach is the wish to identify symptomatic conditions that are treatable with medication. This practice ignores the mediating factors measured on the other axes: personality, stressors, and functional level. The result of one-dimensional diagnosis is one-dimensional therapy.

Environmental Reductionism in Psychiatry

Environmental reductionism is a problem associated with the practice of psychotherapy. Psychotherapists favor environmentalist theories because they seem to provide a more hopeful prognosis. If the primary roots of psychological symptoms lie in childhood, then addressing negative early experiences in treatment might reverse these symptoms. If psychopathology is simply the result of learning the wrong things or being exposed to the wrong parents, then providing the new environment of psychotherapy might reverse these effects.

Some psychotherapists resist genetic theories of mental illness on the grounds that heredity implies irreversibility. This conclusion is based on a series of misunderstandings. First, pathology is determined not by single genes but by multiple interacting genes. Second, the mechanisms by which genes affect the mind are complex and indirect. Third, genetic influences on behavior are never independent of the environment. As discussed in Chapter 2, no individual can be adequately described by a genome.

Moreover, even when the variance in a trait is entirely a function of "the genes," the trait can still be dramatically modified by manipulating environmental factors (Meehl 1973). One famous example is phenylketonuria. This inborn error of metabolism causes serious illness beginning at birth that, if untreated, leads inevitably to severe mental retardation. Yet, although its etiology is entirely due to a defect in a single gene, phenylketonuria can be treated successfully by a simple alteration in diet. This example demonstrates that focusing on genetic factors in psychopathology need not lead to therapeutic nihilism or even to the disparagement of psychotherapy.

Psychotherapists may also be suspicious of genetic constraints on individual development because such constraints contradict their cherished belief in the unlimited nature of human potential (Paris 1973). In contrast, the predisposition–stress model suggests a rather different treatment philosophy. It encourages therapists to be more modest in their expectations of patients. It is concordant with a world view in which each of us must learn to live within the limits of the human condition.

Finally, psychotherapists may be reluctant to consider predispositions to mental disorders if they believe that doing so involves "blaming the victim." Unfortunately, this line of thought implies that there is *always* a victim! Of course, parents *do* make serious mistakes in raising their children, and some life events *do* lie outside our control. Yet, as discussed in Chapters 3, 11, and 15, individuals vary widely in their response to negative events. These findings offer a serious challenge to the environmentalist creed. On the other hand, they need not be used to support the reverse conclusion that patients are responsible for their own difficulties. By taking both nature and nurture into account, we can avoid inappropriate attributions of blame.

Psychotherapists also need to take individual differences into account. When the tailor has only one size of suit, the customer must pay for the adjustments. One of the strengths of the predisposition–stress model is that it addresses individuality while leaving sufficient space for personal responsibility and existential choice. If personality is often the main factor that determines how individuals respond to life's challenges, then therapy must be conducted differently with each patient.

In the future, psychological treatments will be based on more interactive etiological theories. Our present "dynamic formulations" of psychopathology fail to take into account how the same experiences have different effects on individuals with different personality traits.

Let us consider an example of how this principle might be applied in practice.

Beyond Reductionism: The Treatment of Personality Disorders

In recent years, the treatment of psychological symptoms has relied more and more on either drugs or behavioral interventions and less and less on traditional psychodynamic methods of psychotherapy. As a result, the province of the psychotherapist has been steadily shrinking, with long-term therapies coming to be seen as suitable only for patients with Axis II pathology (Gunderson 1985). It seems logical to expect that long-term difficulties must require long-term treatments, which clinical tradition has usually considered to be the treatment of choice for personality disorders.

Yet how effective are these treatments? The earliest study of the treatment of patients with personality disorders was carried out at the Menninger Clinic in the 1950s. The strongest finding was that patients with greater initial ego strength had the best outcome (Kernberg et al. 1972). Yet there was no evidence that taking an "uncovering" approach was more useful than providing supportive therapy (Horwitz 1974). Moreover, many patients in this study remained in treatment for the rest of their lives (R. Wallerstein 1986).

Two fairly recent reports (Monsen et al. 1995; Stevenson and Meares 1992) have suggested that psychodynamic psychotherapy for patients with personality disorders can be effective, at least for selected patients. However, like the Menninger study, neither of these studies used control groups for comparison. As a result, we cannot separate therapeutic effects from naturalistic improvement over time.

Moreover, we do not know whether the patients who undergo long-term therapy are representative of personality disorder patients as a group. Some patients with Axis II pathology are not very interested in psychotherapy. Over half of patients with borderline personality disorder drop out within a few months when offered open-ended treatment (Gunderson et al. 1989), even when they had originally requested it.

Because of their reputation for being hard to treat, patients with personality disorders have been unpopular among psychiatrists (L. Lewis and Appleby 1988). Clinicians who are not committed to long-term psychotherapy often avoid this group entirely. Alternatively, many psychiatrists simply ignore Axis II pathology and focus on comorbid Axis I symptoms that can be managed with drugs.

On the other side of the psychiatric divide, patients with personality disorders are still offered long-term psychotherapy. Most methods continue to be based on the assumption of the primacy of early experience. Thus, borderline personality has been seen as a response to childhood trauma (Herman and van der Kolk 1987). Narcissistic personality has been seen as deriving from failures in parental empathy (Kohut 1970, 1977). Disorders in the anxious cluster have been seen as deriving from the failure of parents to provide secure attachment (Bowlby 1973). These theories all encourage therapists to explore the events of childhood in great detail, in the belief that insight changes intrapsychic structures, and that changes in these structures will lead to changes in behavior.

The assumption that "insight," by itself, is the main factor determining behavioral change in therapy has little empirical support (Lambert and Bergin 1994; Wachtel 1977, 1993). Instead, the psychotherapy research literature shows that many different forms of therapy produce equivalent results (Beutler et al. 1994). The most important element in therapeutic success is a strong alliance with a therapist (Lambert and Bergin 1994).

In the course of this book, I have criticized the doctrine of the primacy of early experience. There may even be negative effects associated with therapeutic methods that relate problems in the present primarily to events in the past. Patients can use childhood experiences to validate their sense of victimization or to rationalize avoiding change. They may also become embroiled in the process of gaining insight into the past and lose sight of issues that need to be addressed in the present. Finally, psychotherapy that holds parents accountable for all of their children's difficulties runs the risk of depriving patients of needed support and contact with family members.

The treatment of the personality disorders provides a particularly good example of the application of predisposition–stress theory to clinical practice. As discussed in Chapter 15, genetic factors are probably involved in the etiology of these conditions. We therefore need to develop methods of treatment that address the role of these heritable traits. Thus far, drugs are of marginal value in this population (Soloff 1993).

However, there is another way for psychotherapists to take biological factors into account.

The treatment of personality disorders involves a process that might be called "working with traits" (Paris 1998). Most of the difficulties experienced by these patients are rooted in rigid and maladaptive personality traits. Although these traits are grounded in biological variations, they have been amplified by a process of social learning. Psychotherapy, which is a new form of social learning, aims to reverse this process. The main obstacle is that once maladaptive interpersonal behavior develops, it tends to be cyclic and self-reinforcing (Wachtel 1994).

The psychotherapy of the personality disorders can focus on making the patient's existing traits more socially adaptive. There are two possible ways by which this can be accomplished. The first involves the modification of maladaptive behavior patterns. A good example is the reduction of impulsivity and affective instability in borderline personality disorder. This aim might be accomplished, as advocated by psychodynamic therapists (e.g., G. Adler 1985), by offering the patient a consistent "holding environment." In this approach, treatment provides a safe haven within which the patient feels understood and cared for.

Alternatively, similar and possibly even more dramatic results might be achieved through specific behavioral interventions. In "dialectical behavior therapy" (Linehan 1993), impulsivity and affective instability are reduced by psychoeducational methods that target these traits, teaching patients how to tolerate dysphoric emotions and how to solve problems instead of acting impulsively.

In a sense, the ultimate goal of any psychotherapy is behavioral modification. Because traits express themselves through behavior, they must be modified through an educational process that requires patients to practice new behaviors in their daily lives. Whether one calls this "working through" or "behavioral rehearsal," the formidable task of unlearning old behaviors and learning new ones is the main reason that psychotherapy can be a lengthy procedure (Wachtel 1977, 1994).

A second mechanism of change involves helping patients to make their traits work better for them. This involves knowing one's personality and learning to capitalize on it. For example, patients can choose environments that are less stressful and that fit their traits better. Thus, a highly introverted person can choose an occupation in which the environment is very predictable and in which he or she can be productive working alone. A highly extraverted person may do best to choose an environment that presents more challenges and risks and that offers a higher level of interaction with other people.

Nevertheless, treatment usually involves a process of unlearning old behaviors and learning new ones. Psychotherapy in the personality disorders therefore requires what might be called a "two-pronged approach" integrating the psychodynamic and behavioral perspectives. Psychodynamic therapists have always taken into account the historical circumstances that originally led to trait amplification and that continue to affect perceptions of current relationships. Understanding these life experiences also increases empathy and communicates the therapist's interest in the patient as a person. Moreover, knowing the historical origins of maladaptive behavior patterns can be useful in demonstrating that such patterns are being anachronistically applied to present situations.

On the other hand, explaining behavior is rarely a sine qua non for change. History is only a first step. As every therapist knows, patients are often at a loss as to how to apply the self-knowledge they gain from treatment. Patients must learn how to modify traits through behavioral change. This usually requires intensive practice in the "laboratory" of the patient's current interpersonal relationships. Most of the work for the therapist involves focusing on maladaptive patterns in the patient's *present* life and working with the patient to develop adaptive alternatives.

This approach also points to a different approach to making dynamic formulations. As discussed in Chapter 4, psychodynamic models will be more complete when they take predispositions into account. Otherwise, they may only create "narratives" that are not adequate historical explanations of psychopathology (Spence 1983). Thus, if childhood events do not really account for the development of personality disorders, therapists need to move beyond formulations suggesting that behavior "X" is caused by experience "Y."

Instead, therapists can take temperamental vulnerability into account and can share this perspective when making "interpretations." For example, we might tell patients that, given their temperament, certain experiences affect them in a more profound way. Our patients need to know that people differ in their sensitivities and that different people process experience in different ways. Therapists applying this approach would describe a patient's temperament, explain how his or her traits interacted with life experiences, and show how these traits led to an amplification process, eventually creating difficulties in the patient's present life.

Let us consider some examples. In impulsive personality disorders, the therapist might tell patients that given their underlying temperament, and given the fact that they were also exposed to models of impulsivity, they responded by developing impulsive behaviors themselves. More specifically, a patient with an impulsive temperament might be told, "Given your naturally active way of dealing with problems, you did not always understand what you were feeling inside, and this made it particularly hard for you to deal with what happened to you. What caused this to be even harder was that there was no one around to show you how to handle your emotions. Even now, you find this difficult and often end up doing things you regret, instead of looking first at how you feel inside, and then figuring out a way to solve a problem."

Similarly, children who are introverted or "slow to warm up" tend to become more withdrawn when stressed, as a result of either parental overprotection or negative life events. In these patients, we might explain that, given their underlying temperament, they reacted to negative experiences by becoming fearful, mistrustful, and withdrawn. More specifically, a patient with anxious traits might be told, "Because of your natural shyness, you were particularly sensitive to rejection and responded to it by withdrawing even further. What made this even harder was that there was no one around who could help you master these feelings. Even now, you often end up avoiding situations that scare you, instead of accepting your feelings and learning how to get past them."

The idea of using temperament in psychotherapy is not new. Some years ago, Burks and Rubinstein (1979), basing their approach on the research of Chess and Thomas (e.g., 1984), suggested that therapists tell their patients about the temperamental origins of their problems and use temperament to help devise solutions to these problems. Burks and Rubinstein also recommended giving patients a temperament scale to help them understand the nature of their vulnerabilities. However, we probably need to know a great deal more about the biological nature of personality traits before making them the basis of a systematic approach to psychotherapy. Yet even on an unsystematic basis, taking temperament into account has useful clinical applications.

Cognitive-behavior therapy is the only form of psychological therapy that consistently uses a predisposition–stress model of psychopathology. For example, Beck (1986) conceptualized depression as resulting from interactions between a constitutional predisposition to lowered mood and life experiences that produce hopelessness and helplessness. Beck and Freeman (1990) later developed a similar model to account for and to treat personality disorders.

Linehan's (1993) treatment model for borderline personality disorder is also based on predisposition–stress theory. Linehan hypothesized that individuals who subsequently develop borderline personality disorder begin life with a constitutional predisposition that she termed "emotional vulnerability." Negative experiences, which Linehan has termed the "invalidating environment," increase affective instability to pathological proportions. The treatment of borderline personality disorder therefore consists of psychoeducational methods that help these patients regulate their emotions so that they can learn how to solve interpersonal problems. This approach may well turn out to be a model for the treatment of many forms of mental disorder.

▨ Summary

The relationship between nature and nurture provides the conceptual basis for an eclectic clinical practice. The most important principle is that patients with the same diagnosis often require different forms of treatment.

Patients are most likely to require biological interventions when their predispositions are so strong that even the mildest of stressors overwhelm them. This is often the case for patients with schizophrenia and patients with severe mood disorders. In patients with milder predispositions, multiple stressors can produce symptoms by overwhelming resilience. This is often the case for patients with mild depressions and anxiety disorders.

Treating symptoms with pharmacological interventions hastens recovery and allows normal coping mechanisms to be reinstituted. However, many depressed and anxious patients can be treated effectively with psychotherapy alone. Ideally, we should offer our patients the facts and give them the choice. In most cases, combined methods of treatment are the best way to address predisposing and stressing factors in psychopathology. There is some advantage to being a medical practitioner, since the same clinician can offer both psychopharmacology and psychotherapy.

Clinicians should never prescribe medication mechanically, but instead should consider the life stressors, as well as the personality traits, that elicit and maintain symptoms in patients. Similarly, when we prescribe psychotherapy, we can frame the patient's history against a background of individual differences in temperament and personality. Understanding personality traits can be crucial in the prevention of chronicity.

Finally, a predisposition–stress model leads to a different *philosophy* of treatment. When clinicians take predispositions into account, their goals for patients are much more likely to be realistic and pragmatic.

17

Preventive and Research Implications

Nature, Nurture, and Prevention

Clinicians have always been interested in interventions to protect people against mental illness before it starts. However, in order to develop a rational strategy for prevention, we need accurate etiological models of the illnesses we want to prevent.

In the 1960s, there was a great burst of enthusiasm for the idea of a preventive psychiatry. Unfortunately, the ideas behind the community psychiatry movement were based on strong environmentalist assumptions. To consider one example, Caplan (1961) suggested that providing children with a better psychological and social environment could prevent a wide range of adult mental disorders. Unfortunately, these beliefs were based on faith, not facts. Thus far, there is little solid empirical evidence that mental disorders can be effectively prevented through psychosocial interventions.

We have more psychiatrists, more clinical psychologists, and more mental health workers of every kind today than at any other previous point in human history. Yet mental disorders are hardly less common! In fact, as shown by the Epidemiologic Catchment Area study (L. N.

Robins and Regier 1991), several important conditions—depression, substance abuse, and antisocial personality—are now more prevalent than they were a few decades ago.

There could be two explanations for the failures of preventive psychiatry. The first is that we might be able to prevent mental illness by improving social conditions, but we do not yet know how. As discussed in previous chapters, the most likely explanations for recent increases in the prevalence of depression, substance abuse, and antisocial personality involve social stressors. Clinicians have no control over these stressors, most of which are derived from profound forces that are disrupting many of the family and community ties that once provided people with a sense of identity (Paris 1996a). Only the most grandiose therapist could believe that mental health workers can provide anything but the most minimal bulwarks and buffers to counter the juggernaut of modernity.

The second explanation for the failure of preventive psychiatry has practical implications. Past efforts were based on an incorrect model of the etiology of mental illness. In particular, environmentalist theories failed to take into account the genetic factors that could be used to identify high-risk populations in which preventive strategies might be most useful. A preventive psychiatry grounded in a predisposition–stress model of psychopathology could avoid repeating the naive optimism of the past.

A crucial aspect of prevention in the future might involve developing the means to identify biological predispositions prior to the onset of mental disorders. Medicine is on the verge of being able to determine profiles that could define the genetic vulnerability to disease in each individual. Some fear that this information might only frighten and demoralize people. This need not be the case. For example, if we know we are genetically prone to coronary artery disease, we can decide to take particular care of our diet, to exercise, and to avoid smoking. Similarly, if we know we are prone to either essential hypertension or type II diabetes mellitus, we can take action to minimize our risk. Even if we know that we are *not* prone to any of these diseases, we do not have the freedom to lead a totally unhealthy lifestyle, since longevity itself depends on the same environmental risk factors. Although we cannot avoid becoming ill, we can, at the very least, save ourselves a great deal of trouble.

How might we apply these principles to psychiatry? The first step involves accurate measurements of the predispositions to illness (Rutter and Plomin 1997). We already do this, in a rough fashion, by determining whether patients have a family history of a disease. In the future, we can become more precise by carrying out specific biological tests to determine whether an individual is vulnerable to a particular illness. Moreover, taking into account the polygenic nature of most psychiatric illness, we can determine how *quantitatively* strong that predisposition is.

These tests will almost certainly involve measurements of biological markers. Fifty years from now, patients consulting psychiatrists will probably be expected to have routine blood work. In addition, some of the "high-tech" procedures of today, such as positron-emission tomography, could eventually become accessible for the office practitioner.

In the coming decades, understanding the genome may also provide sufficient information to *change* genetic predispositions. Gene therapy for mental disorders may sound like science fiction, but is probably an inevitable development that will become a practical reality sometime in the next century.

In the meantime, genetic information can be used to modify environmental factors, preventing the *expression* of pathogenic genes. For example, the sons of alcoholic fathers are an important target group for early education aimed at preventing the abuse of alcohol or other substances. Similarly, individuals prone to unipolar depression could be an important target population for psychotherapy. Therapists treating this group would carry out psychological interventions designed to teach these individuals to buffer the influence of stressors and to improve the quality of their lives, thus reducing their overall risk for depression.

Disorders arising primarily from biological factors might also be the target of preventive strategies. At present we have few markers for any of these diseases. However, there might be practical advantages to identifying genetic risks early enough.

In the case of schizophrenia, the risk might have to be identified as early as fetal life, since some of the environmental risk factors for this disease develop prior to birth. On the other hand, given the evidence that early treatment of a first episode of schizophrenia leads to a reduction in chronicity (Wyatt 1991), identifying those vulnerable to the disease might allow us to at least offer these individuals more rapid treatment.

One mental disorder about which we have a great deal of genetic information is Alzheimer's disease. Recent evidence (Small et al. 1995) shows that this disease has a familial form, a subtype that is associated with an earlier age at onset. However, even in later-onset, nonfamilial forms of the disease, family histories of dementia are very common (Wise and Gray 1994). There is now evidence that a specific gene, producing apolipoprotein E, is related to both the familial and the sporadic forms of the disease (Corder et al. 1993). This polymorphism is present in about 70% of those who eventually develop Alzheimer's disease.

One might think that, given the prognosis of Alzheimer's disease, people would not want to know about their predispositions. However, treatment might eventually become a practical reality. Gauthier and Poirier (1996) have suggested that if we could develop a method to interfere with the process of beta-amyloid deposition, early identification of cases might reduce the long-term risk for this terrible disease.

In summary, effective strategies for prevention in psychiatry require identifying vulnerable individuals and then targeting any interventions to reach those individuals and populations who are at greatest risk.

Applying the Predisposition–Stress Model to Research on the Etiology of Mental Disorders

Mental disorders arise from a combination of genetic vulnerability and environmental factors. Therefore, in principle, research should aim to determine the relative contributions of predisposition and stress, as well as the interactions between them, in every form of psychiatric illness. Yet few investigations have examined nature and nurture in the same patients. By and large, genetic studies confine themselves to biological factors, and environmental studies confine themselves to psychosocial factors.

The problem is that we cannot usually control for the effects of genetic factors when we study environmental risks, nor can we easily control for the effects of environmental variability when we study genetic risks. The development of genetic epidemiology could bridge this gap. Thus far, much of the research in this discipline depends on twin studies, which are usually limited either to traits in community populations or to disorders with a high enough prevalence to produce sufficient numbers of affected twins. Eventually we will be able to use biological markers to measure specific forms of genetic variability.

At present, even in well-researched illnesses such as schizophrenia, we have no markers to determine precise levels of genetic vulnerability. We must therefore make use of cruder measures, such as the presence of positive family histories. Yet even within these limitations, we could develop research strategies to take gene–environment interactions into account. For example, in studying mood disorders, researchers should determine whether life stresses are more likely to lead to depression in those with a family history of mood disorder or less likely to do so in those without such a history.

Research on the causes of mental disorders should therefore be *multivariate*. The statistical methods of measuring multivariate relationships are widely known, as shown by the frequency of papers in current journals that use regression analyses. These methods allow us to study the percentage of the variance in any disorder accounted for by biological and psychosocial etiological factors. Moreover, research measuring predispositions and stressors in the same samples could help us to overcome the misleading impressions created by univariate associations between risk factors and illness. As long as studies measure genetic or environmental factors separately, we are more easily tempted to read their findings as explanations rather than associations.

Finally, research on nature and nurture in psychiatry could help us to develop a new and better system of classifying mental disorders. Ultimately, psychiatric diagnoses will be based on common predispositions, while measures of stress will remain important as a way of accounting for thresholds of liability for illness.

Conclusions: Integrating Nature and Nurture

I have written this book to offer clinicians a better and more comprehensive model of the probable causes of mental illness. The theory presented here is only a first step toward addressing the question posed in the Introduction: Why, in the presence of the same environmental challenges, do some people develop one type of disorder while others develop an entirely different type?

At our present state of knowledge, this book can provide only a brief sketch of an answer to this question. However, given the current pace and trajectory of psychiatric research, we can expect that the next few decades will yield data to fill in the picture in greater detail. We are just beginning to understand the genetic factors in mental disorders. The study of environmental risk factors is also at an early stage.

Therefore, many of the details described in this book are likely to change. The more successful psychiatric research becomes, the more likely it will be that many of the conclusions presented here will become obsolete. What will probably *not* change, however, is the basic principle that most mental disorders have a genetic component, and that this underlying vulnerability is uncovered by environmental stressors.

Psychiatric theory is undergoing a transition, paralleling changes in other disciplines seeking to understand human behavior. Eventually, the pendulum swing between nature and nurture will be less wild. With time, gene–environment interactions will become the normal frame for thinking about psychopathology. With time, ideas that once seemed overly complex will become truisms.

One word of warning is necessary. Social scientists and mental health workers have long predicted the imminent demise of the nature–nurture dichotomy. In principle, most clinicians have long accepted that "either/or" has to be replaced by "both together." Yet the split between nature and nurture continues.

The political, social, and emotional implications of this debate have led many scientists and clinicians to take one side and ignore the other. A strong commitment to empirical methods in psychiatry could help to counteract these "gut reactions." The ultimate truth concerning scientific questions need not depend on their practical implications. We must be dispassionate about the truth.

Science tells us that nature cannot be understood without nurture, and that nurture cannot be understood without nature. We need to listen to this message, and make it an integral part of our practice.

References

Ackerman N: Treating the Troubled Family. New York, Basic Books, 1966

Adler A: Understanding Human Nature (1927). New York, Fawcett, 1978

Adler G: Borderline Psychopathology and Its Treatment. New York, Jason Aronson, 1985

Akiskal H, Rosenthal TL, Haykal RF: Characterological depressions: clinical and sleep EEG findings separating subaffective dysthymias from character spectrum disorders. Arch Gen Psychiatry 37:777–783, 1980

Alexander F: Psychosomatic Medicine. New York, Norton, 1950

Alnaes R, Torgersen S: Personality and personality disorders predict development and relapses of major depression. Acta Psychiatr Scand 95:336–342, 1997

Amato PR, Booth A: A Generation at Risk. Cambridge, MA, Harvard University Press, 1997

Amato PR, Keith B: Parental divorce and the well-being of children: a meta-analysis. Psychol Bull 110:26–46, 1991

American Psychiatric Association: Diagnostic and Statistical Manual: Mental Disorders. Washington, DC, American Psychiatric Association, 1952

American Psychiatric Association: Diagnostic and Statistical Manual of Mental Disorders, 2nd Edition. Washington, DC, American Psychiatric Association, 1968

American Psychiatric Association: Diagnostic and Statistical Manual of Mental Disorders, 3rd Edition. Washington, DC, American Psychiatric Association, 1980

American Psychiatric Association: Diagnostic and Statistical Manual of Mental Disorders, 3rd Edition, Revised. Washington, DC, American Psychiatric Association, 1987

American Psychiatric Association: Diagnostic and Statistical Manual of Mental Disorders, 4th Edition. Washington, DC, American Psychiatric Association, 1994

Andreasen NC: The Broken Brain. New York, Harper & Row, 1984

Andreasen NC, Rice J, Endicott J, et al: The family history approach to diagnosis: how useful is it? Arch Gen Psychiatry 43:421–429, 1986

Andreasen NC: Creativity and mental illness: prevalence rates in writers and their first-degree relatives. Am J Psychiatry 44:1288–1292, 1987

Arieti S: Interpretation of Schizophrenia, 2nd Edition. New York, Basic Books, 1974

Atkeson BM, Calhoun KS, Resick PA: Victims of rape: repeated assessment of depressive symptoms. J Consult Clin Psychol 50:96–102, 1982

Auden WH: In Memory of Sigmund Freud (1939), in Selected Poems of WH Auden. Edited by Mendelsohn E. New York, Random House, 1979, p 37

Austin MA: The Kaiser-Permanente Women Twins Study data set. Genet Epidemiol 10:519–522, 1993

Baker LA, Cesa IL, Gatz M, et al: Genetic and environmental influences on positive and negative affect: support for a two-factor theory. Psychol Aging 7:158–163, 1992

Baker RA: Hidden Memories. Buffalo, NY, Prometheus Books, 1990

Bandura A: Social Learning Theory. Englewood Cliffs, NJ, Prentice Hall, 1977

Barash D: The Whisperings Within. New York, Harper & Row, 1982

Barkham M, Rees A, Stiles WB, et al: Dose-effect relations in time limited psychotherapy. J Consult Clin Psychol 64:927–935, 1997

Bartlett FC: Remembering: A Study in Experimental and Social Psychology (1932). New York, Cambridge University Press, 1995

Bass E, Davis L: The Courage to Heal. New York, Harper & Row, 1988

Bateson G, Jackson D, Haley J, et al: Towards a theory of schizophrenia. Behav Sci 1:251–256, 1956

Beck AT: Cognitive Therapy and the Emotional Disorders. New York, Basic Books, 1986

Beck AT, Freeman A: Cognitive Therapy of Personality Disorders. New York, Guilford, 1990

Bell JI: Polygenic disease. Curr Opin Genet Dev 3:466–469, 1993

Benedict R: Patterns of Culture (1934). Boston, MA, Houghton Mifflin, 1961

Benjamin J, Patterson C, Greenberg BD, et al: Population and familial association between the D_4 receptor gene and measures of novelty seeking. Nat Genet 12:81–84, 1996

Bergin AE, Garfield SL (eds): Handbook of Psychotherapy and Behavior Change. New York, Wiley, 1994

Bernstein DP, Cohen P, Skodol A, et al: Childhood antecedents of adolescent personality disorders. Am J Psychiatry 153:907–913, 1996

Berretini WH, Ferraro TN, Goldfin LR, et al: A linkage study of bipolar illness. Arch Gen Psychiatry 54:27–35, 1997

Berrios GE: History of the affective disorders, in Handbook of Affective Disorders, 2nd Edition. Edited by Paykel ES. New York, Guilford, 1992, pp 43–56

Bertelsen A, Harvald B, Hauge M: A Danish twin study of manic-depressive disorders. Br J Psychiatry 130:330–351, 1977

Bettelheim B: The Empty Fortress. New York, Free Press, 1967

Beutler LE, Machado PP, Neufeldt SA: Therapist variables, in Handbook of Psychotherapy and Behavior Change. Edited by Bergin AE, Garfield SL. New York, Wiley, 1994, pp 229–269

Biederman J, Faraone SV, Keinan K: Further evidence for family genetic risk factors in attention deficit hyperactivity disorders. Arch Gen Psychiatry 49:728–738, 1992

Biederman J, Faraone SV, Mick E, et al: High risk for attention deficit disorder among children of parents with childhood onset disorder: a pilot study. Am J Psychiatry 152:431–435, 1995a

Biederman J, Milberger S, Faraone SV, et al: Family environment risk factors for attention deficit hyperactivity disorder. Arch Gen Psychiatry 52:464–470, 1995b

Biederman J, Faraone SV, Milberger S, et al: Predictors of persistence and remission of ADHD into adolescence. J Am Acad Child Adolesc Psychiatry 35:343–351, 1996

Bierman AW: Atherosclerosis and other forms of arteriosclerosis, in Harrison's Principles of Internal Medicine, 12th Edition. Edited by Braunwald E, Isselbacher KJ, Wilson JD, et al. New York, McGraw-Hill, 1994, pp 1106–1116

Bilder RM: Neuropsychology and neurophysiology in schizophrenia. Curr Opin Psychiatry 9:57–62, 1996

Billings PR, Beckwith J, Alper JS: The genetic analysis of human behavior: a new era? Soc Sci Med 35:227–38, 1992

Black DW, Andreasen NC: Schizophrenia, schizophreniform disorder, and delusional disorder, in The American Psychiatric Press Textbook of Psychiatry, 2nd Edition. Edited by Hales RE, Yudofsky SC, Talbott JA. Washington, DC, American Psychiatric Press, 1994, pp 411–464

Black DW, Noyes R, Pfohl B: Personality disorders in obsessive-compulsive volunteers, a well comparison group, and their first degree relatives. Am J Psychiatry 150:1226–1232, 1993

Blashfield R, Noyes R, Reich J, et al: Personality disorder traits in generalized anxiety and panic disorder patients. Compr Psychiatry 35:329–334, 1994

Bleuler E: Dementia Praecox, or the Group of Schizophrenias (1911). Translated by Zinker J. New York, International Universities Press, 1950

Blum K, Noble EP, Sheridan PJ: Allelic association of human dopamine D_2 receptor in alcoholism. JAMA 263:2055–2060, 1990

Boas F: General Anthropology. Boston, MA, Heath, 1938

Bohman M, Sigvardsson S: A prospective longitudinal study of children registered for adoption. Acta Psychiatr Scand 61:339–355, 1980

Bohman M, Cloninger CR, von Knorring AL: An adoption study of somatoform disorders, III: cross-fostering analysis and genetic relationship to alcoholism and criminality. Arch Gen Psychiatry 41:871–878, 1984

Bohman M, Cloninger CR, Sigvardsson S: The genetics of alcoholism and related disorders. J Psychiatr Res 21:447–452, 1987

Bolos AM, Dean M, Lucas-Derse S: Population and pedigree studies reveal a lack of association between human dopamine D_2 receptor and alcoholism. JAMA 264:3156–3200, 1990

Bookhamer RS, Meyers R, Schrober C: A five-year follow-up of schizophrenics treated by Rosen's direct analysis, compared with controls. Am J Psychiatry 123:602–604, 1966

Bouchard TJ, Lykken DT, McGue M, et al: Sources of human psychological differences: the Minnesota study of twins reared apart. Science 250:223–228, 1990

Bower GH: Awareness, the unconscious, and repression, in Repression and Dissociation: Implications for Personality Theory, Psychopathology, and Health. Edited by Singer J. Chicago, IL, University of Chicago Press, 1990, pp 209–231

Bowers KS, Hilgard ER: Some complexities in understanding memory, in Hypnosis and Memory. Edited by Pettinati HM. New York, Guilford, 1988, pp 3–17

Bowlby J: Attachment. London, Hogarth Press, 1969

Bowlby J: Separation. London, Hogarth Press, 1973

Bowlby J: Loss. London, Hogarth Press, 1980

Braun MM, Caporaso NE, Page WF, et al: A cohort study of twins and cancer. Cancer Epidemiol Biomarkers Prev 4:469–473, 1994a

Braun MM, Caporaso NE, Page WF, et al: Genetic component of lung cancer: cohort study of twins. Lancet 344:440–443, 1994b

Bray GA: Obesity, in The Genetic Basis of Common Diseases. Edited by King RA, Rotter JI, Motulsky AG. New York, Oxford University Press, 1992, pp 507–528

Brenner MH: Mental Illness and the Economy. Cambridge, MA, Harvard University Press, 1977

Breslau N, Davis GC, Andreski P: Traumatic events and posttraumatic stress disorder in an urban population of young adults. Arch Gen Psychiatry 48:216–222, 1991

Breuer J, Freud S: Studies on hysteria (1893–1895), in Standard Edition of the Complete Psychological Works of Sigmund Freud, Vol 2. Translated and edited by Strachey J. London, Hogarth Press, 1955, pp 1–319

Brewin CR: Scientific status of recovered memories. Br J Psychiatry 169:131–134, 1996

Brown DE: Human Universals. Philadelphia, PA, Temple University Press, 1991

Brown GW, Harris T: Social Origins of Depression. New York, Free Press, 1978

Brown GW, Harris T: Life Events and Illness. New York, Guilford, 1989

Brown GW, Harris T, Hepworth C: Life events and endogenous depression. Arch Gen Psychiatry 51:525–534, 1994

Browne A, Finkelhor D: Impact of child sexual abuse: a review of the literature. Psychol Bull 99:66–77, 1986

Brumberg JJ: Fasting Girls: The Emergence of Anorexia Nervosa as a Modern Disease. Cambridge, MA, Harvard University Press, 1988

Buchsbaum MS, Haier RJ: Psychopathology: biological approaches. Annu Rev Psychology 34:401–430, 1983

Burke W, Motulsky AG: Hypertension, in The Genetic Basis of Common Diseases. Edited by King RA, Rotter JI, Motulsky AG. New York, Oxford University Press, 1992, pp 170–191

Burks J, Rubenstein M: Temperament Styles in Adult Interaction. New York, Brunner/Mazel, 1979

Buss D: The Evolution of Desire. New York, Basic Books, 1994

Butler LD, Duran REF, Jasiukaitis P, et al: Hypnotizability and traumatic experience: a diathesis–stress model of dissociative symptomatology. Am J Psychiatry 153 (suppl):42–63, 1996

Buydens-Branchey L, Branchey MH, Noumair D: Age of alcoholism onset: relation to susceptibility to serotonin precursor availability. Arch Gen Psychiatry 46:231–236, 1989

Cadoret RJ, Stewart MA: An adoption study of attention deficit hyperactivity/ aggression and their relationship to adult antisocial personality. Compr Psychiatry 32:73–82, 1991

Cadoret RJ, Troughton E, O'Gorman TW, et al: An adoption study of genetic and environmental factors in drug abuse. Arch Gen Psychiatry 43:1131–1136, 1986

Cadoret RJ, Yates WR, Troughton E, et al: Adoption study demonstrating two genetic pathways to drug abuse. Arch Gen Psychiatry 52:42–52, 1995a

Cadoret RJ, Yates WR, Troughton E, et al: Genetic environmental interaction in the genesis of aggressivity and conduct disorders. Arch Gen Psychiatry 52:916–924, 1995b

Campbell SB: The socialization and social development of hyperactive children, in Handbook of Developmental Psychopathology. Edited by Lewis M, Miller SM. New York, Plenum, 1990, pp 77–92

Caplan G: Prevention of Mental Disorders in Children. New York, Basic Books, 1961

Cardno AG, McGuffin P: Aetiological theories of schizophrenia. Curr Opin Psychiatry 9:45–49, 1996

Carlson EB: Measuring dissociation with the Dissociative Experiences Scale, in Dissociation: Culture, Mind and Body. Edited by Spiegel D. Washington, DC, American Psychiatric Press, 1994, pp 41–58

Carmelli D, Cardon LR, Fabsitz R: Clustering of hypertension, diabetes, and obesity in adult male twins: same genes or same environments? Am J Hum Genet 55:566–573, 1994a

Carmelli D, Selby JV, Quiroga J, et al: Sixteen-year incidence of ischemic heart disease in the NHLBI twin study: a classification of subjects into high- and low-risk groups. Ann Epidemiol 4:198–204, 1994b

Carmelli D, Robinette D, Fabsitz R: Concordance, discordance, and prevalence of hypertension in World War II veteran twins. J Hypertens 12:323–328, 1994c

Carney RM, Rich MW, Freedland KE: Major depressive disorder predicts cardiac events in patients with coronary artery disease. Psychosom Med 50: 627–633, 1988

Chase-Lansdale PL, Cherlin AJ, Kiernan KE: The long-term effects of parental divorce on the mental health of young adults: a developmental perspective. Child Dev 66:1614–1634, 1995

Chess S, Thomas A: Origins and Evolution of Behavior Disorders. New York, Brunner/Mazel, 1984

Chess S, Thomas A: The New York Longitudinal Study: the young adult periods. Can J Psychiatry 35:557–561, 1990

Childs B, Scriver CR: Age at onset and causes of disease. Perspect Biol Med 29:437–460, 1986

Childs B, Moxon ER, Winkelstein JA: Genetics and infectious disease, in The Genetic Basis of Common Diseases. Edited by King RA, Rotter JI, Motulsky AG. New York, Oxford University Press, 1992, pp 71–91

Chomsky N: Syntactic Structures. The Hague, The Netherlands, Mouton, 1957

Christianson SA: Emotional stress and eyewitness memory: a critical review. Psychol Bull 112:284–309, 1992

Claridge G: The Origins of Mental Illness. London, Blackwell, 1985

Clarke A, Clarke A: Early Experience and Behavior. New York, Free Press, 1979

Cloninger CR: Somatoform and dissociative disorders, in The Medical Basis of Psychiatry. Edited by Winokur G, Clayton PJ. Philadelphia, PA, WB Saunders, 1986, pp 123–151

Cloninger CR: A systematic method for clinical description and classification of personality variants. Arch Gen Psychiatry 44:579–588, 1987

Cloninger CR: Turning point in the design of linkage studies of schizophrenia. Am J Med Genet 54:83–92, 1994

Cloninger CR, Bohman M, Sigvardsson S: Inheritance of alcohol abuse: cross-fostering analysis of adopted men. Arch Gen Psychiatry 38:861–868, 1981

Cloninger CR, Sigvardsson S, Bohman M, et al: Predisposition to petty criminality in Swedish adoptees, II: cross-fostering analysis of gene–environment interactions. Arch Gen Psychiatry 39:1242–1247, 1982

Cloninger CR, Sigvardsson S, von Knorring AL: An adoption study of somatoform disorders, II: identification of two discrete somatoform disorders. Arch Gen Psychiatry 41:863–871, 1984

Cloninger CR, Svrakic DM, Pryzbeck TR: A psychobiological model of temperament and character. Arch Gen Psychiatry 50:975–990, 1993

Coccaro EF, Siever LJ, Klar HM, et al: Serotonergic studies in patients with affective and personality disorders. Arch Gen Psychiatry 46:587–599, 1989

Cohler BJ, Stott FM, Musick JS: Adversity, vulnerability, and resilience: cultural and developmental perspectives, in Developmental Psychopathology, Vol 2: Risk, Disorder, and Adaptation. Edited by Cicchetti D, Cohen DJ. New York, Wiley, 1995, pp 753–800

Collins A: In the Sleep Room. Toronto, Canada, Lester & Orpen Dennys, 1988

Constantino JN: CSF HIAA and family history of antisocial personality disorder in newborns. Am J Psychiatry 154:1771–1773, 1997

Cooper JE, Kendell RE, Gurland BJ: A Comparative Study of Mental Hospital Admissions. Institute of Psychiatry Maudsley Monographs No. 20. London, Oxford University Press, 1972

Corder EH, Saunders AM, Strittmatter WJ, et al: Gene dose of apolipoprotein E type 4 allele and the risk of Alzheimer's disease in late onset families. Science 261:921–923, 1993

Costa PT, McRae RR: From catalog to Murray's needs and the five factor model. J Pers Soc Psychol 55:258–265, 1988

Costa PT, Widiger TA (eds): Personality Disorders and the Five-Factor Model of Personality. Washington, DC, American Psychological Association, 1994

Coyne JC, Whiffen VE: Issues in personality as diathesis for depression: the case of sociotropy–dependency and autonomy–self-criticism. Psychol Bull 118:358–378, 1995

Crews F: Skeptical Engagements. New York, Oxford University Press, 1986

Crews F: The Memory Wars. New York, New York Review of Books, 1995

Cronin A: The Peacock and the Ant. New York, Oxford University Press, 1991

Cross-National Collaborative Group: The changing rate of major depression. JAMA 268:3098–3105, 1992

Crow TJ: Aetiology of schizophrenia: an evolutionary theory. International Clinical Psychopharmacology 10 (suppl 3):49–56, 1995

Crowe RR: An adoption study of antisocial personality. Arch Gen Psychiatry 31:785–791, 1974

Cutrona CE, Cadoret RJ, Suhr JA, et al: Interpersonal variables in the prediction of alcoholism among adoptees: evidence for gene-environment interactions. Compr Psychiatry 35:171–179, 1994

Dar R: Treatment of obsessive-compulsive disorder. Curr Opin Psychiatry 9:125–128, 1996

Dawber TR: The Framingham Study: The Epidemiology of Atherosclerotic Heart Disease. Cambridge, MA, Harvard University Press, 1980

Dean M, Carrington M, O'Brien SJ: Genetic restriction of HIV-1 infection and progression to AIDS by a deletion allele of the CRK5 structural gene. Science 273:5283–5285, 1996

Degler CN: In Search of Human Nature: The Decline and Revival of Darwinism in American Social Thought. New York, Oxford University Press, 1991

DeJong CA, van den Brink M, Harteveld FM, et al: Personality disorders in alcoholics and drug addicts. Compr Psychiatry 34:87–94, 1993

DiNicola VF: Anorexia multiforme: self-starvation in historical and cultural context. Transcultural Psychiatric Research Review 27:165–196, 1990

Dollard J, Miller NE: Personality and Psychotherapy. New York, McGraw-Hill, 1950

Dunn J, Plomin R: Separate Lives: Why Siblings Are So Different. New York, Basic Books, 1990

Durkheim E: On Suicide. Translated by Simpson G. New York, Free Press, 1951

Eaton WW: The Sociology of Mental Disorders, 2nd Edition. New York, Praeger, 1986

Ebstein RP, Novick O, Umansky R, et al: Dopamine receptor (D4R) exone III polymorphism associated with the human personality trait of novelty seeking. Nat Genet 12:78–80, 1996

Egeland JA, Hostetter AM: Amish Study, I: affective disorders among the Amish. Am J Psychiatry 140:56–61, 1976

Eisenberg L: The social construction of the human brain. Am J Psychiatry 152:1563–1575, 1995

Elkin I, Shea T, Watkins JT, et al: National Institute of Mental Health Treatment of Depression Collaborative Research Program: general effectiveness of treatments. Arch Gen Psychiatry 46:971–982, 1989

Ellenberger H: The Discovery of the Unconscious. New York, Basic Books, 1970

Elston RC, Stewart J: A general model for the genetic analysis of pedigree data. Hum Hered 21:523–542, 1971

Engel GL: The clinical application of the biopsychosocial model. Am J Psychiatry 137:535–544, 1980

Erlenmeyer-Kirling L, Squires-Wheeler E, Adamo UH: Psychoses and cluster A personality disorders in offspring of schizophrenic parents at 23 years of follow-up. Arch Gen Psychiatry 52:857–865, 1995

Esman AH: "Sexual abuse," pathogenesis, and enlightened skepticism. Am J Psychiatry 151:1101–1103, 1994

Eysenck HJ: Handbook of Abnormal Psychology. London, Pitman, 1973

Eysenck HJ: Culture and personality abnormalities, in Culture and Psychopathology. Edited by Al-Issa I. Baltimore, MD, University Park Press, 1982, pp 277–308

Eysenck HJ: Genetic and environmental contributions to individual differences: the three major dimensions of personality. J Pers 58:245–261, 1991

Fairbairn WR: Psychoanalytic Studies of the Personality. London, Routledge Kegan-Paul, 1952

Falconer DS: Introduction to Quantitative Genetics. Essex, UK, Longman, 1989

Falloon IRH, Boyd JL, McGill CW: Family Care of Schizophrenia. New York, Guilford, 1984

Fancher RT: Cultures of Healing. New York, WH Freeman, 1995

Faraone SV, Tsuang MT: Methods in psychiatric genetics, in Textbook in Psychiatric Epidemiology. Edited by Tsuang MT, Tohen M, Zahner GEP. New York, Wiley-Liss, 1995, pp 81–134

Faraone SV, Biederman WJ, Keenan J: Separation of attention-deficit disorder and conduct disorder: evidence from a family genetic study of American child psychiatric patients. Psychol Med 21:109–121, 1991

Farvelli C, Pallanti S: Recent life events and panic disorder. Am J Psychiatry 146:622–626, 1989

Fava M, Alpert JE, Borus JS, et al: Patterns of personality disorder comorbidity in early onset versus late-onset major depression. Am J Psychiatry 153: 1308–1312, 1996

Feighner JP, Robins E, Guze SB, et al: Diagnostic criteria for use in psychiatric research. Arch Gen Psychiatry 26:57–63, 1972

Feinlieb M: History of the genetic epidemiology of coronary heart disease. Prog Clin Biol Res 147:1–10, 1984

Feldman RB, Zelkowitz P, Weiss M, et al: A comparison of the families of borderline personality disorder mothers and the families of other personality disorder mothers. Compr Psychiatry 36:157–163, 1995

Femina DD, Yeager CA, Lewis DO: Child abuse: adolescent record vs. adult recall. Child Abuse Negl 145:227–231, 1990

Fergusson DM, Lynskey MT, Horwood J: Childhood sexual abuse and psychiatric disorder in young adulthood, I: prevalence of sexual abuse and factors associated with sexual abuse. J Am Acad Child Adolesc Psychiatry 34: 1355–1364, 1996a

Fergusson DM, Lynskey MT, Horwood J: Childhood sexual abuse and psychiatric disorder in young adulthood, II: psychiatric outcomes of childhood sexual abuse. J Am Acad Child Adolesc Psychiatry 34:1365–1374, 1996b

Fichter MM, Noegel R: Concordance for bulimia nervosa in twins. Int J Eat Disord 9:15–34, 1990

Field LL: Insulin-dependent diabetes mellitus: a model for the study of multifactorial disorders. Am J Hum Genet 43:793–798, 1988

Finkelhor D: The trauma of child sexual abuse: two models, in Lasting Effects of Child Sexual Abuse. Edited by Wyatt GE, Powell GJ. Beverly Hills, CA, Sage, 1988, pp 61–82

Finkelhor D, Hotaling G, Lewis IA, et al: Sexual abuse in a national survey of adult men and women: prevalence characteristics and risk factors. Child Abuse Negl 14:19–28, 1990

Fisher HE: Anatomy of Love. New York, Fawcett Columbine, 1992

Fisher S, Greenberg R: Freud Scientifically Appraised: Testing the Theories and Therapy. New York, Wiley, 1996

Flach F: The resilience hypothesis and posttraumatic stress disorder, in Posttraumatic Stress Disorder: Etiology, Phenomenology, and Treatment. Edited by Wolf ME, Mosnaim AD. Washington, DC, American Psychiatric Press, 1990, pp 37–45

Folstein SE, Piven J: Etiology of autism: genetic influences. Pediatrics 87 (suppl):767–773, 1991

Fonagy P, Leigh T, Steele M, et al: The relation of attachment status, psychiatric classification, and response to psychotherapy. J Consult Clin Psychol 64:22–31, 1996

Fontana A, Rosenheck R: Posttraumatic stress disorder among Vietnam theatre veterans: a causal model of etiology in a community sample. J Nerv Ment Dis 182:677–684, 1994

Foster DW: Diabetes mellitus, in Harrison's Principles of Internal Medicine, 12th Edition. Edited by Braunwald E, Isselbacher KJ, Wilson JD, et al. New York, McGraw-Hill, 1994, pp 1979–2000

Fox R: Kinship and Marriage. New York, Cambridge University Press, 1993

Frank E, Anderson B, Reynolds CF, et al: Life events and the Research Diagnostic Criteria endogenous subtype. Arch Gen Psychiatry 51:519–524, 1994

Frank J, Frank JB: Persuasion and Healing: A Comparative Study of Psychotherapy. Baltimore, MD, Johns Hopkins University Press, 1991

Freeman D: Margaret Mead and Samoa. Cambridge, MA, Harvard University Press, 1983

Freud S: The aetiology of hysteria (1896), in The Standard Edition of the Psychological Works of Sigmund Freud, Vol 3. Translated and edited by Strachey J. London, Hogarth Press, 1962, pp 191–224

Freud S: The interpretation of dreams (1900), in The Standard Edition of the Psychological Works of Sigmund Freud, Vols 4 and 5. Translated and edited by Strachey J. London, Hogarth Press, 1953, pp 1–678

Freud S: Civilized sexual morality and modern nervous diseases (1908), in The Standard Edition of the Psychological Works of Sigmund Freud, Vol 9. Translated and edited by Strachey J. London, Hogarth Press, 1959, pp 177–204

Freud S: Notes on a case of an obsessional neurosis (1909a), in The Standard Edition of the Psychological Works of Sigmund Freud, Vol 10. Translated and edited by Strachey J. London, Hogarth Press, 1955, pp 151–320

Freud S: Analysis of a phobia in a five-year-old boy (1909b), in The Standard Edition of the Psychological Works of Sigmund Freud, Vol 10. Translated and edited by Strachey J. London, Hogarth Press, 1955, pp 1–149

Freud S: Fragment of an analysis of a case of hysteria (1909c), in The Standard Edition of the Psychological Works of Sigmund Freud, Vol 7. Translated and edited by Strachey J. London, Hogarth Press, 1953, pp 7–134

Freud S: The future prospects of psychoanalytic therapy (1910), in The Standard Edition of the Psychological Works of Sigmund Freud, Vol 11. Translated and edited by Strachey J. London, Hogarth Press, 1957, pp 139–151

Freud S: Totem and taboo (1913), in The Standard Edition of the Psychological Works of Sigmund Freud, Vol 13. Translated and edited by Strachey J. London, Hogarth Press, 1958, pp 1–164

Freud S: Introductory lectures on psycho-analysis (1916), in The Standard Edition of the Psychological Works of Sigmund Freud, Vol 15. Translated and edited by Strachey J. London, Hogarth Press, 1963, pp 1–239

Freud S: The psychogenesis of a case of homosexuality in a woman (1920), in The Standard Edition of the Psychological Works of Sigmund Freud, Vol 18. Translated and edited by Strachey J. London, Hogarth Press, 1955, pp 145–174

Freud S: Civilization and its discontents (1930), in The Standard Edition of the Psychological Works of Sigmund Freud, Vol 21. Translated and edited by Strachey J. London, Hogarth Press, 1961, pp 21–134

Freud S: New introductory lectures on psychoanalysis (1933), in The Standard Edition of the Psychological Works of Sigmund Freud, Vol 22. Translated and edited by Strachey J. London, Hogarth Press, 1964, pp 3–182

Friedman M: The Pathology of Coronary Artery Disease. New York, McGraw-Hill, 1969

Fromm E: Escape From Freedom (1940). New York, Fawcett, 1978

Fromm-Reichmann F: Principles of Intensive Psychotherapy. Chicago, IL, University of Chicago Press, 1950

Fromm-Reichmann F: Psychotherapy of schizophrenia. Am J Psychiatry 111: 410–415, 1954

Fromuth ME: The relationship of childhood sexual abuse with later psychological and sexual adjustment in a sample of college women. Child Abuse Negl 10:5–15, 1986

Gabbard G: Psychodynamics in Clinical Practice: The DSM-IV Edition. Washington, DC, American Psychiatric Press, 1994

Gabbard G, Goodwin DW: Integrating biological and psychological perspectives, in American Psychiatric Press Review of Psychiatry, Vol 15. Edited by Dickstein LJ, Riba MB, Oldham JM. Washington, DC, American Psychiatric Press, 1996, pp 527–540

Gardner H: Frames of Mind: The Theory of Multiple Intelligences. New York, Basic Books, 1985

Garfield SL: Research on client variables in psychotherapy, in Handbook of Psychotherapy and Behavior Change. Edited by Bergin AE, Garfield SL. New York, Wiley, 1994, pp 190–228

Garfinkel PE, Kennedy SH, Kaplan AS: Views on classification and diagnosis of eating disorders. Can J Psychiatry 40:445–456, 1995

Garmezy N, Masten AS: Chronic adversities, in Child and Adolescent Psychiatry: Modern Approaches, 3rd Edition. Edited by Rutter M, Hersov L. London, Blackwell, 1994, pp 191–208

Garner DM, Garfinkel PE: The eating attitudes test: an index of the symptoms of anorexia nervosa. Psychol Med 9:273–279, 1979

Garner DM, Garfinkel PE: Socio-cultural factors in the development of anorexia nervosa. Psychol Med 10:647–656, 1980

Garner DM, Garfinkel PE: Handbook of Psychotherapy for Anorexia Nervosa and Bulimia. New York, Guilford, 1985

Garner DM, Olmsted MP, Polivy J, et al: Comparisons between weight-preoccupied women and anorexia nervosa. Psychosom Med 46:255–266, 1984

Gatz M, Pedersen NL, Plomin R, et al: Importance of shared genes and shared environments for symptoms of depression in older adults. J Abnorm Psychol 101:701–708, 1992

Gauthier S, Poirier J: Effects on decline or deterioration, in Alzheimer's Disease: From Molecular Biology to Therapy. Edited by Becker R, Giacobini E. Boston, MA, Birkhauser, 1996, pp 375–406

Geertz C: Local Knowledge. New York, Basic Books, 1983

Gellner E: The Psychoanalytic Movement, 2nd Edition. London, Fontana, 1993

Gershon ES: Genetics, in Manic Depressive Illness. Edited by Goodwin FK, Jamison KR. New York, Oxford University Press, 1990, pp 373–401

Gershon ES, Nurnberger JI: Bipolar illness, in Review of Psychiatry, Vol 14. Edited by Oldham JM, Riba MB. Washington, DC, American Psychiatric Press, 1995, pp 405–424

Gianoulakis C, Krishnan B, Thavundayil J: Enhanced sensitivity of pituitary beta-endorphin to ethanol in subjects at high risk for alcoholism. Arch Gen Psychiatry 53:250–257, 1996

Gold JM, Weinberger DR: Cognitive deficits and the neurobiology of schizophrenia. Curr Opin Neurobiol 5:225–230, 1995

Goldberg D, Huxley P: Common Mental Disorders: A Bio-Social Model. London, Tavistock/Routledge, 1992

Goldbloom DS, Garfinkel PE: The serotonin hypothesis of bulimia nervosa: theory and evidence. Can J Psychiatry 35:741–744, 1990

Goldstein JL: Genetic aspects of disease, in Harrison's Principles of Internal Medicine, 12th Edition. Edited by Braunwald E, Isselbacher KJ, Wilson JD, et al. New York, McGraw-Hill, 1994, pp 339–349

Goldstein MG, Niaura R: Psychological factors affecting physical condition: coronary artery disease and sudden death. Psychosomatics 33:134–145, 1992

Goodwin DW: Alcoholism and genetics: the sins of the fathers. Arch Gen Psychiatry 42:171–174, 1985

Goodwin FK, Jamison KR: Manic-Depressive Illness. New York, Oxford University Press, 1990

Goodwin DW, Warnock JK: Alcoholism: a family disease, in Clinical Textbook of Addictive Disorders. Edited by Frances RJ, Miller SI. New York, Guilford, 1991, pp 485–500

Gottesman I: Schizophrenia Genesis. New York, Freeman, 1991

Gould SJ: The Mismeasure of Man. New York, Norton, 1981

Gould SJ: Eight Little Piggies. New York, Norton, 1993

Gould SJ, Lewontin RC: The spandrels of San Marco and the Panglossian paradigm: a critique of the adaptationist programme. Proceedings of the Royal Society of London 205:581–598, 1979

Green H: I Never Promised You a Rose Garden. New York, Holt, Rinehart, & Winston, 1964

Grinker RR: Psychiatry rushes madly in all directions. Arch Gen Psychiatry 10:228–237, 1964

Gronberg H, Damber L, Damber JE: Studies of genetic factors in prostate cancer in a twin population. J Urol 152:1484–1487, 1994

Grosskurth P: Melanie Klein: Her World and Her Work. New York, Knopf, 1986

Grunbaum A: The Foundations of Psychoanalysis: A Philosophical Critique. Berkeley, CA, University of California Press, 1984

Gull W: Proceedings of the Clinical Society of London. BMJ 1:527–529, 1873

Gunderson JG: Conceptual risks of the Axis I–II division, in Biological Response Styles: Clinical Implications. Edited by Klar H, Siever LJ. Washington, DC, American Psychiatric Press, 1985, pp 81–95

Gunderson JG, Phillips KA: A current view of the interface between borderline personality disorder and depression. Am J Psychiatry 148:967–975, 1991

Gunderson JG, Frank AF, Ronningstam EF, et al: Early discontinuance of borderline patients from psychotherapy. J Nerv Ment Dis 177:38–42, 1989

Guntrip H: Schizoid Phenomena, Object Relations, and the Self. New York, International Universities Press, 1969

Gutheil TG: True or false memories of sexual abuse: a forensic psychiatric view. Psychiatric Annals 23:527–531, 1993

Guzder J, Paris J, Zelkowitz P, et al: Risk factors for borderline personality disorder in children. J Am Acad Child Adolesc Psychiatry 35:26–33, 1996

Guze S: Why Psychiatry is a Medical Specialty. New York, Oxford University Press, 1992

Haastrup S, Thomsen K: The social backgrounds of young addicts as elicited in interviews with their parents. Acta Psychiatr Scand 48:146–173, 1972

Halbreich U, Piletz J, Halarais A: Influence of gonadal hormones on neurotransmitters, receptors, cognition, and mood. Clin Neuropharmacol 15 (suppl):590A–591A, 1992

Hale R: The Rise and Crisis of Psychoanalysis in the United States. New York, Oxford University Press, 1995

Hales RE, Zatzick DF: What is PTSD? Am J Psychiatry 154:143–145, 1997

Halmi KA: Eating disorders, in The American Psychiatric Press Textbook of Psychiatry, 2nd Edition. Edited by Hales RE, Yudofsky SC, Talbott JA. Washington, DC, American Psychiatric Press, 1994, pp 857–875

Hamilton M: A rating scale for depression. J Neurol Neurosurg Psychiatry 23:51–56, 1960

Harding CM, Brooks GW, Ashikaga T, et al: Vermont Longitudinal Study of persons with severe mental illness Am J Psychiatry 143:727–735, 1987

Harlow HF: The nature of love. Am Psychol 13:673–680, 1958

Harris M: Cultural Materialism. New York, Random House, 1979

Head SB, Baker JD, Williamson DA: Family environment characteristics and dependent personality disorder. J Personal Disord 5:256–263, 1991

Heath AC: What can we learn about the determinants of psychopathology and substance abuse from studies of normal twins? in Twins as a Tool of Behavioral Genetics. Edited by Bouchard TJ, Propping P. New York, Wiley, 1993, pp 273–285

Heath AC, Bucholz PA, Madden PAF, et al: Genetic and environmental contributions to alcohol dependence risk in a national twin sample: consistency of findings in women and men. Psychol Med 27:1381–1396, 1997

Hechtman L: Genetic factors in attention deficit disorder. J Psychiatry Neurosci 19:193–201, 1994

Helzer JE, Canino GJ (eds): Alcoholism in North America, Europe, and Asia. New York, Oxford University Press, 1992

Helzer JE, Robins LN, Davis DH: Antecedents of narcotic use and addiction. Drug Alcohol Depend 3:183–190, 1976

Helzer JE, Robins LBN, Wishe E: Depression in Vietnam veterans and civilian controls. Am J Psychiatry 136:526–529, 1979

Herman J: Father-Daughter Incest. Cambridge, MA, Harvard University Press, 1981

Herman J: Trauma and Recovery. New York, Basic Books, 1992

Herman JL, van der Kolk BA: Traumatic antecedents of borderline personality disorder, in Psychological Trauma. Edited by van der Kolk BA. Washington, DC, American Psychiatric Press, 1987, pp 111–126

Herman JL, Perry JC, van der Kolk BA: Childhood trauma in borderline personality disorder. Am J Psychiatry 146:490–495, 1989

Herrero ME, Hechtman L, Weiss G: Antisocial disorders in hyperactive subjects from childhood to adulthood. Am J Orthopsychiatry 64:510–521, 1992

Hesselbrock VM: Genetic determinants of alcohol subtypes, in The Genetics of Alcoholism. Edited by Begleiter H, Kissin B. New York, Oxford University Press, 1995, pp 122–135

Hetherington EM, Cox M, Cox R: Long-term effects of divorce and remarriage on the adjustment of children. Journal of the American Academy of Child Psychiatry 24:518–530, 1985

Hoch PH, Cattell JP, Strahl MD, et al: The course and outcome of pseudoneurotic schizophrenia. Am J Psychiatry 119:106–115, 1962

Hogarty GE, Anderson C, Reiss D, et al: Family psychoeducation, social skills training and maintenance chemotherapy in the aftercare treatment of schizophrenia. Arch Gen Psychiatry 48:340–347, 1991

Hogarty GE, Greenwald D, Ulrich RF, et al: Three-year trials of personal therapy among schizophrenic patients living with or independent of family, II: effects of adjustment of patients. Am J Psychiatry 154:1514–1525, 1997

Holland AJ, Sicotte N, Tresure J: Anorexia nervosa: evidence for a genetic basis. J Psychosom Res 32:561–571, 1988

Hollander E, Simeon D, Gorman JM: Anxiety disorders, in The American Psychiatric Press Textbook of Psychiatry, 2nd Edition. Edited by Hales RE, Yudofsky SC, Talbott JA. Washington, DC, American Psychiatric Press, 1994, pp 496–564

Hollingshead A, Redlich F: Social Class and Mental Illness. New York, Wiley, 1958

Holmes D: The evidence for repression: an examination of sixty years of research, in Repression and Dissociation: Implications for Personality Theory, Psychopathology, and Health. Edited by Singer J. Chicago, IL, University of Chicago Press, 1990, pp 85–102

Holzman PS: On the trail of the genetics and pathophysiology of schizophrenia. Psychiatry 59:117–127, 1996

Hopkins PN, Williajs RTR, Kuida H: Family history as an independent risk factor for incident coronary artery disease in a high-risk cohort. Journal of Chronic Diseases 62:703–707, 1986

Horney K: The Neurotic Personality of Our Time. New York, Norton, 1940

Horowitz M: Stress-response syndromes, in International Handbook of Traumatic Stress Syndromes. Edited by Wilson JP, Raphael B. New York, Plenum, 1993, pp 49–60

Horwitz L: Clinical Prediction in Psychotherapy. New York, Jason Aronson, 1974

Howard KI, Kopta AM, Krause MS, et al: The dose-effect relationship to psychotherapy. Am Psychol 41:159–164, 1986

Hsu LKG, Chesler BE, Santhouse R: Bulimia nervosa in eleven sets of twins. Int J Eat Disord 9:275–282, 1990

Hull C: Essentials of Behavior (1951). New York, Greenwood, 1974

Hwu HG, Yeh EK, Change LY: Prevalence of psychiatric disorders in Taiwan defined by the Chinese Diagnostic Interview Schedule. Acta Psychiatr Scand 79:136–147, 1989

Irwin HJ: Traumatic childhood events, perceived availability of emotional support, and the development of dissociative tendencies. Child Abuse Negl 20:709–722, 1996

Jablensky A, Sartorius N, Ernberg G, et al: Schizophrenia: manifestations, incidence and course in different cultures. Psychol Med Monogr Suppl 20, 1992

James W: The Principles of Psychology (1895). Cambridge, MA, Harvard University Press, 1981

Janet P: The Major Symptoms of Hysteria. New York, Macmillan, 1907

Jang KL, Livesley WJ, Vernon PA: Alcohol and drug problems: a multivariate behavioral genetic analysis of co-morbidity. Addiction 90:1213–1221, 1995

Jang KL, Livesley WJ, Vernon PA, et al: Heritability of personality traits: a twin study. Acta Psychiatr Scand 94:438–444, 1996

Jang K, Paris J, Zweig-Frank H, et al: A twin study of dissociative experience. J Nerv Ment Dis 186:345–351, 1998

Jefferson JW, Greist JH: Mood disorders, in The American Psychiatric Press Textbook of Psychiatry, 2nd Edition. Edited by Hales RE, Yudofsky SC, Talbott JA. Washington, DC, American Psychiatric Press, 1994, pp 465–494

Jellinek EM: The Disease Concept of Alcoholism. New Haven, CT, Hillhouse, 1960

Jenike MA: Obsessive-compulsive disorder, in Comprehensive Textbook of Psychiatry, 5th Edition. Edited by Kaplan H, Freedman A, Sadock B. Baltimore, MD, Williams & Wilkins, 1995, pp 1218–1226

Jensen PSD, Hoagwood K: The book of names: DSM-IV in context. Dev Psychopathol 9:231–250, 1997

Johnson C, Connors ME: The Etiology and Treatment of Bulimia Nervosa. New York, Basic Books, 1987

Jones D, Fox MM, Babigian MM: Epidemiology of anorexia nervosa in Monroe County. Psychosom Med 42:551–558, 1980

Judd FK, Burrows GD: Anxiety disorders and their relationship to depression, in Handbook of Affective Disorders, 2nd Edition. Edited by Paykel ES. New York, Guilford, 1992, pp 77–87

Jung CG: Psychological Types. New York, Harcourt Brace, 1921

Kagan J: Galen's Prophecy. New York, Basic Books, 1994

Kandel ER: A new intellectual framework for psychiatry. Am J Psychiatry 155:457–469, 1998

Kanner L: Autistic disturbances of affective contact. Nervous Child 2:217–250, 1943

Kaufman C, Grunebaum H, Cohler B, et al: Superkids: competent children of schizophrenic mothers. Am J Psychiatry 136:1398–1402, 1979

Kendell RE: The stability of psychiatric diagnoses. Br J Psychiatry 114:611–626, 1974

Kendler KS: Genetic epidemiology in psychiatry: taking both genes and environment seriously. Arch Gen Psychiatry 52:895–899, 1995

Kendler KS: Parenting: a genetic epidemiological perspective. Am J Psychiatry 153:11–20, 1996

Kendler KS: The diagnostic validity of melancholic major depression in a population-based sample of female twins. Arch Gen Psychiatry 54:299–304, 1997a

Kendler KS: Social support: a genetic epidemiological analysis. Am J Psychiatry 154:1398–1404, 1997b

Kendler KS, Eaves LJ: Models for the joint effect of genotype and environment on liability to psychiatric illness. Am J Psychiatry 143:279–289, 1986

Kendler KS, Gardner CO: Boundaries of major depression: an evaluation of DSM-IV criteria. Am J Psychiatry 155:172–177, 1998

Kendler KS, Gruenberg AM: An independent analysis of the Danish Adoption Study of Schizophrenia. Arch Gen Psychiatry 41:555–564, 1984

Kendler KS, Prescott CA: Cannabis use, abuse, and dependence in a population-based sample of female twins. Am J Psychiatry 155:1016–1022, 1998

Kendler KS, Gruenberg AM, Strauss JJ: An independent analysis of the Copenhagen sample of the Danish Adoption Study of Schizophrenia, II: the relationship between schizotypal personality disorder and schizophrenia. Arch Gen Psychiatry 38:983–984, 1981

Kendler KS, Masterson CC, Ungaro R, et al: A family history study of schizophrenia-related personality disorders. Am J Psychiatry 143:424–428, 1984

Kendler KS, Heath A, Martin NG: Symptoms of anxiety and symptoms of depression: same genes, different environment? Arch Gen Psychiatry 44:451–457, 1987

Kendler KS, Maclean C, Neale MC, et al: The genetic epidemiology of bulimia nervosa. Am J Psychiatry 148:1627–1637, 1991

Kendler KS, Heath AC, Neale MC, et al: A population-based twin study of alcoholism in women. JAMA 268:1877–1882, 1992a

Kendler KS, Neale MC, Kessler RC: Generalized anxiety disorder in women: a population-based twin study. Arch Gen Psychiatry 49:267–272, 1992b

Kendler KS, Neale MC, Kessler RC: The genetic epidemiology of phobias in women: the interrelationship of agoraphobia, social phobia, situational phobia, and simple phobia. Arch Gen Psychiatry 49:273–280, 1992c

Kendler KS, Neale MC, Kessler RC, et al: Familial influences on the clinical characteristics of major depression: a twin study. Acta Psychiatr Scand 86:371–378, 1992d

Kendler KS, Neale M, Kessler R, et al: A twin study of recent life events and difficulties. Arch Gen Psychiatry 50:789–796, 1993a

Kendler KS, Neale M, Kessler R: Panic disorder in women: a population-based twin study. Psychol Med 23:397–406, 1993b

Kendler KS, Neale M, Kessler R, et al: A longitudinal twin study of personality and major depression in women. Arch Gen Psychiatry 50:853–862, 1993c

Kendler KS, Neale MC, Kessler RC, et al: A test of the equal-environment assumption in twin studies of psychiatric illness. Behav Genet 23:21–27, 1993d

Kendler KS, Kessler RC, Neale MC, et al: The prediction of major depression in women: toward an integrated, etiologic model. Am J Psychiatry 150:1139–1148, 1993e

Kendler KS, Neale MC, Heath AC, et al: A twin-family study of alcoholism in women. Am J Psychiatry 151:707–715, 1994

Kendler KS, Neale M, Kessler R: The structure of the genetic and environmental risk factors for six major psychiatric disorders in women. Arch Gen Psychiatry 52:464–470, 1995a

Kendler KS, Kessler RC, Walters EE: Stressful life events, genetic liability, and onset of an episode of major depression in women. Am J Psychiatry 152:833–842, 1995b

Kendler KS, Eaves LJ, Walters EE, et al: The identification and validation of distinct depressive syndromes in a population-based sample of female twins. Arch Gen Psychiatry 53:391–399, 1996

Kennedy JL: Schizophrenia genetics: the quest for an anchor. Am J Psychiatry 153:1513–1514, 1996

Kernberg OF: Borderline Conditions and Pathological Narcissism. New York, Jason Aronson, 1975

Kernberg OF, Coyne L, Appelbaum A, et al: Final report of the Menninger Psychotherapy Research Project. Bull Menninger Clin 36:1–275, 1972

Kerr M, Tremblay RE, Pagaini L, et al: Boys' behavioral inhibition and the risk of later delinquency. Arch Gen Psychiatry 54:809–816, 1997

Kessler RC, McGonagle KA, Nelson CB, et al: Lifetime and 12-month prevalence of DSM-III-R psychiatric disorders in the United States. Arch Gen Psychiatry 51:8–19, 1994

Kettner B: Combat strain and subsequent mental health. Acta Psychiatr Scand Suppl 230:1–112, 1972

Kety SS, Rosenthal D, Wender PH: Mental illness in the biological and adoptive families of adopted individuals who have become schizophrenic, in Genetic Research in Psychiatry. Edited by Fieve R, Rosenthal D, Brill H. Baltimore, MD, Johns Hopkins University Press, 1975, pp 147–165

Kety SS, Wender PW, Jacobsen B, et al: Prewar factors in combat-related post-traumatic stress disorder: structural equation modeling with a national sample of female and male Vietnam veterans. J Consult Clin Psychol 64:520–531, 1996

Kevles DJ: In the Name of Eugenics. New York, Knopf, 1985

Keys A, Aravanis C, Blackburn HW, et al: Epidemiological studies related to coronary heart disease. Acta Med Scand Suppl 460:1–392, 1966

Khantzian EJ: Self-medication hypothesis of addictive disorders. Am J Psychiatry 142:1259–1264, 1985

Kihlstrom JF: One hundred years of hysteria, in Dissociation: Clinical and Theoretical Perspectives. Edited by Lynn SJ, Rhue JW. New York, Guilford, 1994, pp 365–394

King RA, Rotter JI, Motulsky AG: The approach to genetic bases of common diseases, in The Genetic Basis of Common Diseases. Edited by King RA, Rotter JI, Motulsky AG. New York, Oxford University Press, 1992, pp 3–18

Kirmayer LJ: Cultural aspects of dissociation, in Dissociation: Culture, Mind, and Body. Edited by Spiegel D. Washington, DC, American Psychiatric Press, 1994a, pp 91–122

Kirmayer LJ: Is the concept of mental disorder culturally relative? in Controversial Issues in Mental Health. Edited by Kirk SA, Einbinder S. Boston, MA, Allyn & Bacon, 1994b, pp 1–20

Kirmayer LJ: Confusion of the senses: implications of ethnocultural variations in somatoform and dissociative disorders for PTSD, in Ethnocultural Aspects of Posttraumatic Stress Disorder. Edited by Marsella AJ, Friedman MJ, Gerrity ET, et al. Washington, DC, American Psychological Association, 1996, pp 131–163

Kirmayer LJ, Robbins JM, Paris J: Somatoform disorders: personality and the social matrix of somatic distress. J Abnorm Psychol 103:125–136, 1994a

Kirmayer LJ, Young A, Robbins JM: Symptom attribution in cultural perspective. Can J Psychiatry 39:584–595, 1994b

Kitcher P: Vaulting Ambition: Sociobiology and the Quest for Human Nature. Cambridge, MA, MIT Press, 1985

Klein DF, Rabkin JG, Gorman JM: Etiological and pathophysiological inference from the pharmacological treatment of anxiety disorders, in Anxiety and the Anxiety Disorders. Edited by Tuma AH, Maser JD. Hillsdale, NJ, Lawrence Erlbaum, 1985

Klein G: Psychoanalytic theory. New York, International Universities Press, 1976

Klein M: Envy and Gratitude. New York, International Universities Press, 1946

Klerman G: Historical perspectives on contemporary schools of psychopathology, in Contemporary Psychopathology: Towards the DSM-IV. Edited by Millon T, Klerman G. New York, Guilford, 1986, pp 3–28

Klerman GL, Weissman MM: Increasing rates of depression. JAMA 261:2229–2235, 1989

Klerman GL, DiMascio A, Weissman MM, et al: Treatment of depression by drugs and psychotherapy. Am J Psychiatry 131:186–191, 1974

Knapp PH, Mathe AA: Psychophysiological aspects of bronchial asthma: a review, in Bronchial Asthma: Mechanisms and Therapeutics. Edited by Weiss EB, Segal MS, Stein M. Boston, MA, Little, Brown, 1985, pp 914–931

Knowles JA, Weissman MM: Panic disorder and agoraphobia, in Review of Psychiatry, Vol 14. Edited by Oldham JM, Riba MB. Washington, DC, American Psychiatric Press, 1995, pp 383–404

Knudson AG: Hereditary cancer: two hits revisited. J Cancer Res Clin Oncol 122:135–140, 1996

Kocsis JH, Sutton BM, Frances AJ: Long-term follow-up of chronic depression treated with imipramine. J Clin Psychiatry 52:56–59, 1991

Kohut H: The Analysis of the Self. New York, International Universities Press, 1970

Kohut H: The Restoration of the Self. New York, International Universities Press, 1977

Konner M: The Tangled Wing. New York, Harper & Row, 1983

Kopta SM, Howard KI, Lowry JL, et al: Patterns of symptomatic recovery in psychotherapy. J Consult Clin Psychol 62:1009–1016, 1994

Kraemer HC, Kazdin AE, Offord DR: Coming to terms with the terms of risk. Arch Gen Psychiatry 54:337–345, 1997

Kraepelin E: Dementia Praecox and Paraphrenia. Translated by Barclay M, edited by Robertson GM. Edinburgh, Scotland, E & S Livingstone, 1919

Krueger RF, Caspi A, Moffitt TE, et al: Personality traits are differentially linked to mental disorders: a multitrait–multidiagnosis study of an adolescent birth cohort. J Abnorm Psychol 105:299–312, 1996

Kuhn T: The Structure of Scientific Revolutions. Chicago, IL, University of Chicago Press, 1970

Kumar D, Gemayel NS, Deapen D, et al: North American twins with IDDM. Diabetes 42:1351–1363, 1993

Laing RD: The Politics of Experience. New York, Penguin, 1967

Lambert MJ, Bergin AE: The effectiveness of psychotherapy, in Handbook of Psychotherapy and Behavior Change. Edited by Bergin AE, Garfield SL. New York, Wiley, 1994, pp 143–189

Laufer RS, Gallops MS, Frey-Wouters E: War stress and trauma. J Health Soc Behav 25:65–85, 1984

Laurence JR, Perry C: Hypnotically created memory among highly hypnotizable subjects. Science 222:523–524, 1983

Lazarus RS, Folkman S: Stress, Appraisal and Coping. New York, Springer, 1984

Lee KA, Vaillant GE, Torrey WC, et al: A 50-year prospective study of the psychological sequelae of World War II combat. Am J Psychiatry 152:516–522, 1995

Leff JP: Psychiatry Around the Globe. London, Gaskell, 1988

Leff JP, Sartorius N, Jablensky A, et al: The International Pilot Study of Schizophrenia. Psychol Med 22:131–145, 1992

Lehmann H: Affective disorders: clinical features, in Comprehensive Textbook of Psychiatry, 3rd Edition. Edited by Kaplan H, Freedman A, Sadock B. Baltimore, MD, Williams & Wilkins, 1985, pp 786–810

Leighton DC, Harding JS, Macklin DB: The Character of Danger: Psychiatric Symptoms in Selected Communities. New York, Basic Books, 1963

Lesch KP, Bengel D, Heils A, et al: Association of anxiety-related traits with a polymorphism in the serotonin transporter gene regulatory region. Science 274:1527–1531, 1996

Levins R, Lewontin RC: The Dialectical Biologist. Cambridge, MA, Harvard University Press, 1985

Levinson DF, Mahtani MM, Nancarrow DJ, et al: Genome scan of schizophrenia. Am J Psychiatry 155:741–750, 1998

Levi-Strauss C: The Elementary Structures of Kinship. Boston, MA, Beacon, 1969

Levy F, Hay DA, McStephen M, et al: Attention-deficit disorder: a category or a continuum? Genetic analysis of a large-scale twin study. J Am Acad Child Adolesc Psychiatry 36:737–744, 1997

Lewinsohn PM, Mischel W, Chaplin W, et al: Social competence and depression: the role of illusory self-perceptions. J Abnorm Psychol 89:203–212, 1980

Lewis A: The survival of hysteria. Psychol Med 5:9–12, 1975

Lewis L, Appleby L: Personality disorder: the patients psychiatrists dislike. Br J Psychiatry 153:44–49, 1988

Lewis M: Altering Fate. New York, Guilford, 1997

Lewontin RC: Biology as Ideology: The Doctrine of DNA. New York, Harper Collins, 1992

Lewontin RC, Rose S, Kamin LJ: Not in Our Genes: Biology, Ideology and Human Nature. New York, Pantheon, 1985

Lidz T, Blatt S: Critique of the Danish-American studies of biological and adoptive relatives of adoptees who became schizophrenic. Am J Psychiatry 140:426–435, 1983

Lidz T, Fleck S: Schizophrenia and The Family. New York, International Universities Press, 1985

Linehan MM: Cognitive Behavioral Therapy of Borderline Personality Disorder. New York, Guilford, 1993

Links PS, Steiner M, Offord DR: Characteristics of borderline personality disorder: a Canadian study. Can J Psychiatry 33:336–340, 1988a

Links PS, Steiner B, Huxley G: The occurrence of borderline personality disorder in the families of borderline patients. J Personal Disord 2:14–20, 1988b

Lipowski Z: Psychiatry: mindless or brainless, both or neither? Can J Psychiatry 34:249–254, 1989

Litman RE, Torrey EF, Hommer DW: A quantitative analysis of smooth pursuit eye tracking in monozygotic twins discordant for schizophrenia. Arch Gen Psychiatry 54:417–428, 1997

Littlefield JW: Genes, chromosomes, and cancer. J Pediatr 104:489–494, 1984

Livesley WJ, Jang K, Schroeder ML, et al: Genetic and environmental factors in personality dimensions. Am J Psychiatry 150:1826–1831, 1993

Locke J: Some Thoughts Concerning Education (1693). Cambridge, UK, Cambridge University Press, 1892

Loeber R, Green SM, Keenan K, et al: Which boys will fare worse? Early predictors of the onset of conduct disorder in a six-year longitudinal study. J Am Acad Child Adolesc Psychiatry 34:499–509, 1995

Loftus E: Eyewitness Testimony. Cambridge, MA, Harvard University Press, 1979

Loftus EF: The reality of repressed memories. Am Psychol 48:518–537, 1993

Loranger AW, Sartori N, Andreoli A, et al: The International Personality Disorder Examination. Arch Gen Psychiatry 51:215–224, 1994

Lteif GN, Mavissakalian MR: Life events and panic disorder/agoraphobia. Compr Psychiatry 36:118–122, 1995

Luborsky L, Crits-Christoph P: Understanding Transference: The Core Conflict Relationship Theme Method. New York, Basic Books, 1990

Lumeng L, Murphy JM, McBride WJ, et al: Genetic influences on alcohol preference in animals, in The Genetics of Alcoholism. Edited by Begleiter H, Kissin B. New York, Oxford University Press, 1995, pp 165–201

Lykken D, Tellegen A: Happiness is a stochastic phenomenon. Psychological Science 7:186–189, 1996

Lykken DT, McGue M, Tellegen A, et al: Emergenesis: genetic traits which may not run in families. Am Psychol 47:1565–1577, 1992

Lyons MJ: A twin study of self-reported criminal behavior, in Genetics of Criminal and Antisocial Behavior. Edited by Bock GR, Goode JA. Chichester, UK, John Wiley, 1996, pp 1–75

Lyons MJ, Goldberg J, Eisen SA, et al: Do genes influence exposure to trauma? A twin study of combat. Am J Med Genet 48:22–27, 1993

Lyons MJ, True WR, Eisen SA, et al: Differential heritability of adult and juvenile antisocial traits. Arch Gen Psychiatry 52:916–924, 1995

Lyons MJ, Eisen SA, Goldberg J, et al: A registry-based twin study of depression in men. Arch Gen Psychiatry 55:468–472, 1998

MacDonald MJ: Speculation on the evolution of insulin-dependent diabetes genes. Metabolism 37:1182–1184, 1988

Main M, Hesse E: The insecure/disorganized attachment pattern in infancy: precursors and sequelae, in Attachment in the Preschool Years: Theory, Research, Intervention. Edited by Greenberg M, Ciccheti P, Cummings EM. Chicago, IL, University of Chicago Press, 1991, pp 161–184

Malinovsky-Rummell R, Hansen DJ: Long-term consequences of physical abuse. Psychol Bull 114:68–79, 1993

Manuzza S, Klein RG, Bessler A, et al: Adult psychiatric status of hyperactive boys grown up. Am J Psychiatry 155:493–498, 1998

Marcus J, Hans SL, Auerbach JG, et al: Children at risk for schizophrenia: the Jerusalem infant development study. Arch Gen Psychiatry 50:797–809, 1993

Marenberg ME, Risch N, Berkman LF, et al: Genetic susceptibility to death from coronary heart disease in a study of twins. N Engl J Med 330:1041–1046, 1994

Martin B, Hoffman JA: Conduct disorders, in Handbook of Developmental Psychopathology. Edited by Lewis M, Miller SM. New York, Plenum, 1990, pp 109–118

Maser JD, Cloninger CR (eds): Comorbidity of Anxiety and Depression. Washington, DC, American Psychiatric Press, 1990

Masse LC, Tremblay RE: Behavior of boys in kindergarten and the onset of substance use during adolescence. Arch Gen Psychiatry 54:62–68, 1996

Masson J: The Assault on Truth. New York, Penguin, 1984

Masten AS, Coatsworth JD: Competence, resilience, and psychopathology, in Developmental Psychopathology, Vol 2: Risk, Disorder, and Adaptation. Edited by Cicchetti D, Cohen DJ. New York, Wiley, 1995, pp 715–752

Matsuda A, Kuzuya T: Diabetic twins in Japan. Diabetes Res Clin Pract 24 (suppl):S63–S67, 1994

Maughan B, Rutter M: Retrospective reporting of childhood adversity. J Personal Disord 11:4–18, 1997

May PRA: The Treatment of Schizophrenia. New York, Science House, 1970

Mayr E: The Growth of Biological Thought. Cambridge, MA, Harvard University Press, 1982

Maziade M, Caron C, Coté R, et al: Extreme temperament and diagnosis: a study in a psychiatric sample of consecutive children. Arch Gen Psychiatry 47:477–484, 1990

Maziade M, Roy MA, Martinez M, et al: Negative, psychoticism, and disorganized dimensions in patients with familial schizophrenia or bipolar disorder: continuity and discontinuity between the major psychoses. Am J Psychiatry 152:1458–1463, 1995

Maziade M, Bissonnette L, Rouillard E, et al: 6p24–22 region and major psychoses in the Eastern Quebec population. Am J Med Genet 74:311–318, 1997a

Maziade M, Martinez M, Rodrigue C, et al: Childhood/early adolescence-onset and adult-onset schizophrenia: heterogeneity at the dopamine D_3 receptor gene. Br J Psychiatry 170:27–30, 1997b

McBride P, Anderson GM: Autism research: bringing together approaches to pull apart the disorder. Arch Gen Psychiatry 53:980–982, 1996

McFadden ER: Asthma, in Harrison's Principles of Internal Medicine, 11th Edition. Edited by Braunwald E, Isselbacher KJ, Petersdorf RG, et al. New York, McGraw-Hill, 1987, pp 1060–1065

McFarlane AC: Vulnerability to post-traumatic stress disorder, in Posttraumatic Stress Disorder: Etiology, Phenomenology, and Treatment. Edited by Wolf ME, Mosnaim AD. Washington, DC, American Psychiatric Press, 1990, pp 4–20

McFarlane AC: PTSD: synthesis of research and clinical studies, in International Handbook of Traumatic Stress Syndromes. Edited by Wilson JP, Raphael B. New York, Plenum, 1993, pp 421–429

McFarlane AC: The aetiology of post-traumatic morbidity: predisposing, precipitating, and perpetuating factors. Br J Psychiatry 154:221–228, 1996

McGlashan T: The prediction of outcome in chronic schizophrenia. Arch Gen Psychiatry 43:167–176, 1986

McGlashan T: Schizophrenia: Treatment and Outcome. Washington, DC, American Psychiatric Press, 1989

McGuffin P, Gottesman I: Genetic influences on normal and abnormal development, in Child and Adolescent Psychiatry: Modern Approaches. Edited by Rutter M, Hersov L. Oxford, UK, Blackwell, 1985, pp 17–33

McGuffin P, Thapar A: The genetics of personality disorder. Br J Psychiatry 160:12–23, 1992

McGuffin P, Katz R, Rutherford J: Nature, nurture, and depression: a twin study. Psychol Med 21:329–335, 1991

McGuffin P, Katz R, Watkings S, et al: A hospital-based twin register of the heritability of DSM-IV unipolar depression. Arch Gen Psychiatry 53:129–136, 1996

McGuigan JE: Peptic ulcer and gastritis, in Harrison's Principles of Internal Medicine, 12th Edition. Edited by Braunwald E, Isselbacher KJ, Wilson JD, et al. New York, McGraw-Hill, 1994, pp 1363–1382

McGuire MT, Trossi A: Darwinian Psychiatry. Cambridge, MA, Harvard University Press, 1996

Mead M: Coming of Age in Samoa (1926). New York, Morrow, 1971

Mead M: Male and Female (1950). New York, Morrow, 1975

Mednick S: The Copenhagen high risk project. Schizophr Bull 13:485–495, 1987

Mednick SA, Gabrieli WF, Hutchings B: Genetic influences in criminal convictions. Science 224:891–894, 1984

Mednick S, Machon RA, Huttunen MO: Adult schizophrenia following prenatal exposure to an influenza epidemic. Arch Gen Psychiatry 45:189–192, 1988

Meehl PE: Specific genetic etiology, psychodynamics, and therapeutic nihilism, in Psychodiagnosis: Selected Papers. New York, Norton, 1973

Meehl PE: Toward an integrated theory of schizotaxa, schizotypy, and schizophrenia. J Personal Disord 4:1–99, 1990

Mendelewicz J, Rainer JD: Adoption study supporting genetic transmission in manic-depressive illness. Nature 268:327–329, 1977

Menninger K: The Vital Balance. New York, Peter Smith, 1963

Merskey H: The Analysis of Hysteria, 2nd Edition. London, Gaskell, 1995

Meyer-Williams L: Recall of childhood trauma: a prospective study of women's memories of child sexual abuse. J Consult Clin Psychol 62:1167–1176, 1994

Meyers DA, Marsh DG: Allergy and asthma, in The Genetic Basis of Common Diseases. Edited by King RA, Rotter JI, Motulsky AG. New York, Oxford University Press, 1992, pp 130–149

Midgley JP, Matthew AG, Greenwood CMT, et al: Effect of reduced dietary sodium on blood pressure: a meta-analysis of randomized control trials. JAMA 275:1590–1597, 1996

Miller A: Prisoners of Childhood. New York, Basic Books, 1981

Miller A: Thou Shalt Not Be Aware. New York, Farrar, Strauss, & Giroux, 1984

Millon T: Modern Psychopathology. Philadelphia, PA, WB Saunders, 1969

Millon T, Davis R: Personality Disorders: DSM-IV and Beyond. New York, Wiley, 1995

Mills CW: The Power Elite. New York, Oxford University Press, 1955

Minuchin S, Rosman BL, Baker L: Psychosomatic Families: anorexia nervosa in context. Cambridge, MA, Harvard University Press, 1978

Mirsky IA: Physiological, psychological, and social determinants in the etiology of duodenal ulcer. American Journal of Digestive Diseases 3:285–290, 1958

Monroe SM, Simons AD: Diathesis-stress theories in the context of life stress research. Psychol Bull 110:406–425, 1991

Monsen JT, Odland T, Faugli A, et al: Personality disorders and psychosocial changes after intensive psychotherapy: a prospective follow-up study of an outpatient psychotherapy project, 5 years after end of treatment. Scand J Psychol 36:256–268, 1995

Moos RH, Moos BS: Family Environment Scale: Manual. Palo Alto, CA, Consulting Psychologists Press, 1986

Mora GL: Historical and theoretical trends in psychiatry, in Comprehensive Textbook of Psychiatry, 2nd Edition. Edited by Freedman A, Kaplan H, Sadock B. Baltimore, MD, Williams & Wilkins, 1975, pp 1–75

Motulsky AG, Brunzell JD: The genetics of coronary atherosclerosis, in The Genetic Basis of Common Diseases. Edited by King RA, Rotter JI, Motulsky AG. New York, Oxford University Press, 1992, pp 150–169

Mulder RT, Beautrais AL, Joyce PR, et al: Relationship between dissociation, childhood sexual abuse, childhood physical abuse, and mental illness in a general population sample. Am J Psychiatry 155:806–811, 1998

Muncie WS: Psychobiology and Psychiatry. St Louis, MO, CV Mosby, 1939

Murdock GP: Outline of World Cultures. New Haven, CT, Human Relations Area Files, 1975

Murphy HBM: Comparative Psychiatry. New York, Springer, 1982

Murray RM: Neurodevelopmental schizophrenia: the rediscovery of dementia praecox. Br J Psychiatry 165 (suppl 25):6–12, 1994

Nandi DN, Ajmany S, Ganguli G: Psychiatric disorders in a rural community in West Bengal. Indian J Psychiatry 17:87–89, 1975

Nandi DN, Banerjee G, Nandi S, et al: Is hysteria on the wane? Br J Psychiatry 160:87–91, 1992

Nash MR, Hulsely TL, Sexton MC, et al: Long-term effects of childhood sexual abuse: perceived family environment, psychopathology, and dissociation. J Consult Clin Psychol 61:276–283, 1993

Nesse R, Williams GC: Why We Get Sick. New York, Random House, 1994

Newman SC, Bland RC: Life events and the 1-year prevalence of major depressive episode, generalized anxiety disorder, and panic disorder in a community sample. Compr Psychiatry 35:76–82, 1994

Nieminen MN, Kaprio J, Kosenvuo M: A population-based study of bronchial asthma in adult twin pairs. Chest 100:70–75, 1991

Nigg JT, Goldsmith HH: Genetics of personality disorders: perspectives from personality and psychopathology research. Psychol Bull 115:346–380, 1994

Nigg JT, Goldsmith HH: Developmental psychopathology, personality, and temperament: reflections on recent behavioral genetics research. Human Biology 70:383–408, 1998

Nurnberger JL, Gershon ES: Genetics, in Handbook of Affective Disorders, 2nd Edition. Edited by Paykel ES. New York, Guilford, 1992, pp 131–148

Ofshe R, Watters E: Making Monsters: False Memories, Psychotherapy, and Sexual Hysteria. New York, Scribner, 1994

Ogata SN, Silk KR, Goodrich S: Childhood sexual and physical abuse in adult patients with borderline personality disorder. Am J Psychiatry 147:1008–1013, 1990a

Ogata SN, Silk KR, Goodrich S: The childhood experience of the borderline patient, in Family Environment and Borderline Personality Disorder. Edited by Links PS. Washington, DC, American Psychiatric Press, 1990b, pp 87–103

Orne MT, Whitehouse WG, Dinges DF, et al: Reconstructing memory through hypnosis: forensic and clinical implications, in Hypnosis and Memory. Edited by Pettinati HM. New York, Guilford, 1988, pp 21–54

Paris J: Psychiatry and ideology. Canadian Psychiatric Association Journal 18:147–151, 1973

Paris J: The Oedipus complex: a critical re-examination. Canadian Psychiatric Association Journal 21:173–179, 1976

Paris J: Family theory and character pathology. Int J Family Psychiatry 3:475–485, 1983

Paris J: Personality disorders: a biopsychosocial model. J Personal Disord 7:255–264, 1993

Paris J: Borderline Personality Disorder: A Multidimensional Approach. Washington, DC, American Psychiatric Press, 1994

Paris J: Social Factors in the Personality Disorders. New York, Cambridge University Press, 1996a

Paris J: A critical review of recovered memories in psychotherapy, I: trauma and memory. Can J Psychiatry 41:201–205, 1996b

Paris J: a critical review of recovered memories in psychotherapy, II: trauma and therapy. Can J Psychiatry 41:206–210, 1996c

Paris J: Dissociative symptoms, dissociative disorders, and transcultural psychiatry. Transcultural Psychiatry Research Review 33:55–68, 1996d

Paris J: Antisocial and borderline personality: two separate disorders or two aspects of the same psychopathology? Compr Psychiatry 38:237–242, 1997

Paris J: Working With Traits: Psychotherapy in the Personality Disorders. Northvale, NJ, Jason Aronson, 1998

Paris J: Anxious traits, anxious attachment, and anxious cluster personality disorders. Harv Rev Psychiatry 6:142–148, 1998

Paris J, Zweig-Frank H, Guzder J: Psychological risk factors for borderline personality disorder in female patients. Compr Psychiatry 35:301–305, 1994a

Paris J, Zweig-Frank H, Guzder J: Risk factors for borderline personality in male outpatients. J Nerv Ment Dis 182:375–380, 1994b

Parker G: Parental Overprotection: A Risk Factor in Psychosocial Development. New York, Grune & Stratton, 1983

Parker G: Early environment, in Handbook of Affective Disorders, 2nd Edition. Edited by Paykel ES. New York, Guilford, 1992, pp 171–194

Parsons T: Social Theory and Modern Society. New York, Free Press, 1967

Patience DA, McGuire RJ, Scott AIF, et al: The Edinburgh Primary Care Depression Study: personality disorder and outcome. Br J Psychiatry 167:324–330, 1995

Paykel ES, Cooper Z: Life events, in Handbook of Affective Disorders, 2nd Edition. Edited by Paykel ES. New York, Guilford, 1992, pp 149–170

Pepper CM, Klein DN, Anderson RL, et al: DSM-III-R Axis II comorbidity in dysthymia and major depression. Am J Psychiatry 152:239–247, 1995

Peterson WL: Helicobacter pylori and peptic ulcer disease. N Engl J Med 324: 1043–1048, 1991

Pettinati HM: Hypnosis and memory: integrative summary and future directions, in Hypnosis and Memory. Edited by Pettinati HM. New York, Guilford, 1988, pp 277–292

Pfohl B, Coryell W, Zimmerman M, et al: DSM-III personality disorders: diagnostic overlap and internal consistency of individual DSM-III criteria. Compr Psychiatry 27:21–34, 1986

Phillips KA, Gunderson JG, Hirschfeld RMA: A review of the depressive personality. Am J Psychiatry 147:830–837, 1990

Pihl RO, Peterson J: Inherited predisposition to alcoholism. J Abnorm Psychol 99:291–301, 1990

Pike A, Plomin R: Importance of nonshared environmental factors for childhood and adolescent psychopathology. J Am Acad Child Adolesc Psychiatry 35:560–570, 1996

Pike A, Reiss D, Hetherington EM, et al: Family environment and adolescent depressive symptoms and antisocial behavior: a multivariate genetic analysis. Dev Psychol 32:590–603, 1996

Pinker S: The Language Instinct. New York, Harper Collins, 1994

Pinker S: How The Mind Works. New York, Norton, 1997

Piper A: Hoax and Reality: The Bizarre World Of Multiple Personality Disorder. Northvale, NJ, Jason Aronson, 1997

Piven J, Palmer P, Jacobi D, et al: Broader autism phenotype: evidence from a family history study of multiple-incidence families. Am J Psychiatry 154: 185–190, 1997

Plomin R: Genetics and Experience. Thousand Oaks, CA, Sage, 1994a

Plomin R: Genetic research and identification of environmental influences. J Child Psychol Psychiatry 35:817–834, 1994b

Plomin R, Bergeman CS: The nature of nurture: genetic influence on "environmental" measures. Behav Brain Sci 14:373–427, 1991

Plomin R, Rutter M: Child development, molecular genetics, and what to do with genes once they are found. Child Dev (in press)

Plomin R, Chuiper HM, Loehlin JC: Behavior genetics and personality, in Handbook of Personality Theory and Research. Edited by Pervin LA. New York, Guilford, 1990a, pp 226–240

Plomin R, Nitz K, Rowe DC: Behavioral genetics and aggressive behavior in children, in Handbook of Developmental Psychopathology. Edited by Lewis M, Miller SM. New York, Plenum, 1990b, pp 199–134

Plomin R, DeFries JC, McClearn GE, et al: Behavioral Genetics, 3rd Edition. New York, WH Freeman, 1997

Polivy J, Herman CP: Dieting and bingeing: a causal analysis. Am Psychol 40:193–201, 1985

Pope HG, Hudson JI: Can memories of childhood sexual abuse be repressed? Psychol Med 25:121–126, 1995

Popper CW, Steingard RJ: Disorders first diagnosed in infancy, childhood, or adolescence, in The American Psychiatric Press Textbook of Psychiatry, 2nd Edition. Edited by Hales RE, Yudofsky SC, Talbott JA. Washington, DC, American Psychiatric Press, 1994, pp 729–832

Popper K: Conjectures and Refutations. New York, Harper Torch, 1968

Post RM: Transduction of psychosocial stress into the neurobiology of recurrent affective disorder. Am J Psychiatry 149:999–1010, 1992

Prince R, Tseng-Laroche F: Culture-bound syndromes and international disease classification. Culture, Medicine, and Psychiatry 11:1–49, 1990

Raff MC: Death wish. The Sciences 36:36–40, 1996

Rahe RH: Stress and psychiatry, in Comprehensive Textbook of Psychiatry, 5th Edition. Edited by Kaplan H, Freedman A, Sadock B. Baltimore, MD, Williams & Wilkins, 1995, pp 1545–1559

Rapaport JL (ed): Obsessive-Compulsive Disorder in Children and Adolescents. Washington, DC, American Psychiatric Press, 1989

Rastam M: Anorexia nervosa in 51 Swedish adolescents: premorbid problems and comorbidity. J Am Acad Child Adolesc Psychiatry 31:819–829, 1992

Rastam M, Gillberg G: The family background in anorexia nervosa. J Am Acad Child Adolesc Psychiatry 30:283–289, 1991

Regier DA, Burke JD: Epidemiology, in Comprehensive Textbook of Psychiatry, 6th Edition. Edited by Kaplan HI, Sadock BJ. Baltimore, MD, Williams and Wilkins, 1995, pp 377–396

Reich T: A golden age for psychiatric genetics. Lecture at Allan Memorial Institute, Montreal, Canada, March 28, 1996

Reiss D, Plomin R, Hetherington EM: Genetics and psychiatry: an unheralded window on the environment. Am J Psychiatry 149:147–155, 1992

Reiss D, Hetherington EM, Howe GW, et al: Genetic questions for environmental studies: differential parenting and psychopathology in adolescence. Arch Gen Psychiatry 52:925–936, 1995

Rende RD, Plomin R, Reiss D, et al: Genetic and environmental influences on depressive symptomatology in adolescence: individual differences and extreme scores. J Child Psychol Psychiatry 34:1387–1398, 1993

Rind B, Tromovitch P, Bauserman R: A meta-analytic examination of assumed properties of child sexual abuse using college samples. Psychol Bull 124: 22–53, 1998

Riso LP, Klein DN, Ferro T, et al: Understanding the comorbidity between early onset dysthymia and cluster B personality disorders: a family study. Am J Psychiatry 153:900–906, 1996

Robins E, Guze SB: Establishment of diagnostic validity in psychiatric illness: its application to schizophrenia. Am J Psychiatry 126:107–111, 1970

Robins LN: Deviant Children Grown Up. Baltimore, MD, Williams & Wilkins, 1966

Robins LN, Regier DA (eds): Psychiatric Disorders in America. New York, Free Press, 1991

Robins LN, Helzer JE, Croughan D: National Institute of Mental Health Diagnostic Interview Schedule. Arch Gen Psychiatry 38:381–389, 1981

Robins LN, Schoenberg SP, Holmes SJ: Early home environment and retrospective recall: a test for concordance between siblings with and without psychiatric disorders. Am J Orthopsychiatry 55:27–41, 1985

Rodgers B: Pathways between parental divorce and adult depression. J Child Psychol Psychiatry 35:1289–1308, 1994

Romans SE, Martin JL, Anderson JC, et al: Factors that mediate between childhood sexual abuse and adult outcome. Psychol Med 25:127–142, 1995

Rosen J: Direct Analysis. New York, Grune & Stratton, 1953

Rosenbaum JF, Biederman J, Bolduc-Murphy EA, et al: Behavioral inhibition in childhood: a risk factor for anxiety disorders. Harv Rev Psychiatry 1:2–17, 1993

Rosenthal D: The Genain Quadruplets. New York, Basic Books, 1968

Rosenthal D: Genetics of Psychopathology. New York, McGraw-Hill, 1971

Rothbart MK, Ahadi SA: Temperament and the development of personality. J Abnorm Psychol 103:55–66, 1994

Rotter JI, Vadheim CM, Rimoin DL: Diabetes mellitus, in The Genetic Basis of Common Diseases. Edited by King RA, Rotter JI, Motulsky AG. New York, Oxford University Press, 1992a, pp 413–481

Rotter JI, Shohat T, Petersen GM: Peptic ulcer disease, in The Genetic Basis of Common Diseases. Edited by King RA, Rotter JI, Motulsky AG. New York, Oxford University Press, 1992b, pp 240–278

Rowe DC: Environmental and genetic influences on dimensions of perceived parenting: a twin study. Dev Psychol 17:203–208, 1981

Roy MA, Neale MC, Pedersen NL, et al: A twin study of generalized anxiety disorder and major depression. Psychol Med 25:1037–1049, 1995

Rumantsyev SN: Observations on constitutional resistance to infection. Immunol Today 13:184–187, 1992

Russell D: The Secret Trauma: Incest in the Lives of Girls and Women. New York, Basic Books, 1986

Rutter M: Psychopathology and development: links between childhood and adult life, in Child and Adolescent Psychiatry: Modern Approaches. Edited by Rutter M, Hersov L. Oxford, UK, Blackwell, 1985, pp 720–742

Rutter M: Psychosocial resilience and protective mechanisms. Am J Orthopsychiatry 57:316–331, 1987a

Rutter M: Temperament, personality, and personality development. Br J Psychiatry 150:443–448, 1987b

Rutter M: Pathways from childhood to adult life. J Child Psychol Psychiatry 30:23–51, 1989

Rutter M: Nature, nurture, and psychopathology: a new look at an old topic. Dev Psychopathol 3:125–136, 1991

Rutter M: Mental disorders in childhood and adulthood. Acta Psychiatr Scand 91:73–85, 1995

Rutter M: Nature–nurture integration: the example of antisocial behavior. Am Psychol 52:390–398, 1997

Rutter M, Maughan B: Psychosocial adversities in psychopathology. J Personal Disord 11:19–33, 1997

Rutter M, Plomin R: Opportunities for psychiatry from genetic findings. Br J Psychiatry 171:209–219, 1997

Rutter M, Quinton D: Long-term follow-up of women institutionalized in childhood. British Journal of Developmental Psychology 18:225–234, 1984

Rutter M, Rutter M: Developing Minds: Challenge and Continuity Across the Life Span. New York, Basic Books, 1993

Rutter M, Cox A, Tupling C, et al: Attainment and adjustment in two geographical areas. Br J Psychiatry 126:493–509, 1975

Rutter M, MacDonald A, Le Couteur R, et al: Genetic factors in child psychiatric disorders: II: empirical findings. J Child Psychol Psychiatry 31:39–83, 1990

Rutter M, Dunn J, Plomin R, et al: Integrating nature and nurture: implications of person–environment correlations and interactions for developmental psychopathology. Dev Psychopathol 9:335–364, 1997

Sarafino EP, Goldfedder J: Genetic factors in the presence, severity, and triggers of asthma. Arch Dis Child 73:112–116, 1995

Scarr S: Race, Social Class, and Individual Differences in Intelligence. Hillsdale, NJ, Lawrence Erlbaum, 1981

Scarr S: The construction of family reality. Behav Brain Sci 14:385–386, 1991

Scarr S, McCartney K: How people make their own environments: a theory of genotype-environment effects. Child Dev 54:424–435, 1983

Schacter DL: Searching for Memory. New York, Basic Books, 1996

Scheff TJ: Labelling Madness. New York, Prentice Hall, 1975

Schuckit MA: Biological markers in alcoholism. Prog Neuropsychopharmacol Biol Psychiatry 10:191–199, 1986

Schuckit MA, Smith TL: An 8 year follow-up of 450 sons of alcoholic and control subjects. Arch Gen Psychiatry 53:202–210, 1996

Schwartz CE, Snidman N, Kagan J: Early childhood temperament as a determinant of externalizing behavior in adolescence. Dev Psychopathol 8:527–537, 1996

Searles H: Collected Papers on Schizophrenia and Related Subjects. New York, International Universities Press, 1965

Seeman MV: Schizophrenia, gender, and affect. Can J Psychiatry 41:263–264, 1996

Seeman P, Bzowej NH, Guan HC: Human brain D_1 and D_2 dopamine receptors in Schizophrenia. Neuropsychopharmacology 1:5–15, 1987

Seligman ME: Helplessness. New York, WH Freeman, 1975

Shaffer D: Attention deficit hyperactivity disorder in adults. Am J Psychiatry 151:633–638, 1994

Shapiro T, Emde R: Research on Psychoanalysis: process, development, outcome. New York, International Universities Press, 1994

Shea MT, Pilkonis PA, Beckahm E: Personality disorders and treatment outcome in the NIMH Treatment of Depression Collaborative Research Program. Am J Psychiatry 147:711–718, 1990

Shea MT, Elkin I, Imber SD: Course of depressive symptoms over follow-up. Arch Gen Psychiatry 49:782–787, 1992

Shear MK, Cooper AM, Klerman GL, et al: A psychodynamic model of panic disorder. Am J Psychiatry 150:859–866, 1993

Sherfey MJ: The evolution and nature of female sexuality in relation to psychoanalytic theory. J Am Psychoanal Assoc 14:28–128, 1966

Shields J: Monozygotic Twins Raised Together and Apart. Oxford, UK, Oxford University Press, 1962

Shorter E: From Mind to Body. New York, Free Press, 1994

Shorter E: A History of Psychiatry. New York, Free Press, 1997

Showalter E: Hystories. New York, Columbia University Press, 1996

Siever LJ, Davis KL: A psychobiological perspective on the personality disorders. Am J Psychiatry 148:1647–1658, 1991

Siever LJ, Keefe R, Bernstein DP, et al: Eye tracking impairment in clinically identified patients with schizotypal personality disorder. Am J Psychiatry 147:740–745, 1990

Sigal JJ, Weinfeld M: Trauma and Rebirth: Intergenerational Effects of the Holocaust. New York, Praeger, 1989

Sigvardsson S, von Knorring AL, Bohman M: An adoption study of somatoform disorders, I: the relationship to psychiatric liability. Arch Gen Psychiatry 41: 853–859, 1984

Sigvardsson S, Bohman M, Cloninger R: Replication of the Stockholm adoption study of alcoholism. Arch Gen Psychiatry 53:681–687, 1996

Silberg JL, Rutter ML, Meyer J, et al: Genetic and environmental influences on the covariation between hyperactivity and conduct disturbance in juvenile twins. J Child Psychol Psychiatry 37:803–816, 1996

Silverman JM, Pinkham L, Horvath TB, et al: Affective and impulsive personality disorder traits in the relatives of patients with borderline personality disorder. Am J Psychiatry 148:1378–1385, 1991

Skinner BF: Verbal Behavior. Englewood Cliffs, NJ, Prentice Hall, 1957

Skre I, Onstad S, Torgersen S, et al: A twin study of DSM-III-R anxiety disorders. Acta Psychiatr Scand 88:85–92, 1993

Slutske WS, Heath AC, Dinwiddie SH, et al: Modeling genetic and environmental influences in the etiology of conduct disorder: a study of 2,682 adult twin pairs. J Abnorm Psychol 106:266–279, 1997

Slyper A, Schectman G: Coronary artery disease risk factors from a genetic and developmental perspective. Arch Intern Med 154:633–638, 1994

Small GW, Mazziota JC, Collins MT: Apoliprotein E type 4 allele and cerebral glucose metabolism in relatives at risk for familial Alzheimer disease. JAMA 273:942–947, 1995

Snow CP: The Two Cultures (1958). Cambridge, UK, Cambridge University Press, 1993

Snyder S: The opiate receptor and morphine-like peptides in the brain. Am J Psychiatry 135:645–652, 1978

Soloff PH: Psychopharmacological intervention in borderline personality disorder, in Borderline Personality Disorder: Etiology and Treatment. Edited by Paris J. Washington, DC, American Psychiatric Press, 1993, pp 319–348

Solomon Z, Benbenishty R, Mikulincer M: A follow-up of the Israel casualties of combat stress reaction (battle shock) in the 1982 Lebanon war. Br J Clin Psychol 27:125–135, 1988

Sorensen TIA, Nielsen GG, Andersen PK, et al: Genetic and environmental influences on premature death in adult adoptees. N Engl J Med 318:727–732, 1988

Southwick SM, Yehuda R, Giller EL: Personality disorders in treatment-seeking combat veterans with post-traumatic stress disorder. Am J Psychiatry 150: 1020–1023, 1993

Southwick SM, Morgan A, Nicolau AL, et al: Consistency of memory for combat-related traumatic events in veterans of Operation Desert Storm. Am J Psychiatry 154:173–177, 1997

Spanos NP: Hypnotic behavior: a cognitive social psychological perspective. Research Communications in Psychology, Psychiatry, and Behavior 7:199–213, 1982

Spence D: Narrative Truth and Historical Truth. New York, Norton, 1983

Spence D: Interpretation: a critical perspective, in Interface of Psychoanalysis and Psychology. Edited by Barron JW, Eagle MN, Wolitsky DL. Washington, DC, American Psychological Association, 1992, pp 558–572

Spiegel D: Hypnosis, dissociation, and trauma, in Repression and Dissociation: Implications for Personality Theory, Psychopathology, and Health. Edited by Singer J. Chicago, IL, University of Chicago Press, 1990, pp 121–143

Spiegel D, Cardena E: Disintegrated experience: the dissociative disorders revisited. J Abnorm Psychol 100:366–378, 1991

Srole L: The Midtown Manhattan Longitudinal Study vs. "the mental paradise lost" doctrine. Arch Gen Psychiatry 37:209–221, 1980

Stanley D, Wand RR: Obsessive-compulsive disorder: a review of the cross-cultural literature. Transcultural Psychiatric Research Review 32:103–136, 1995

Stanton AH, Gunderson JG, Knapp PH: Effects of psychotherapy in schizophrenia. Schizophr Bull 10:520–563, 1984

Staudinger UM, Marsiske, Baltes PB: Resilience and reserve capacity in later adulthood: potentials and limits of development across the life span, in Developmental Psychopathology, Vol 2: Risk, Disorder, and Adaptation. Edited by Cicchetti D, Cohen DJ. New York, Wiley, 1995, pp 801–848

Stefanis C, Markidis M, Christodoulou G: Observations of the evolution of the hysterical symptomatology. Br J Psychiatry 128:269–275, 1976

Stehbens WE: The concept of cause in disease. Journal of Chronic Diseases 38:945–950, 1985

Steiger H, Stotland S: Individual and family factors in adolescents with eating disorders and syndromes, in Eating Disorders in Adolescence. Edited by Steinhausen H-C. New York, de Gruyter, 1995, pp 49–68

Steiger H, Liquornik K, Chapman J, et al: Personality and family disturbances in eating disorder patients. Int J Eat Disord 10:501–512, 1991

Steiger H, Jabalpurwala S, Champagne J: Axis II comorbidity and developmental adversity in bulimia nervosa. J Nerv Ment Dis 184:555–560, 1996

Steinberg M: Interviewer's Guide to the Structured Clinical Interview for DSM-IV Dissociative Disorders. Washington, DC, American Psychiatric Press, 1994

Stern D: The Interpersonal World of the Infant. New York, Basic Books, 1985

Stern J, Murphy M, Bass C: Personality disorders in patients with somatization disorder: a controlled study. Br J Psychiatry 363:785–789, 1993

Stevens A, Price J: Evolutionary Psychiatry. London, Routledge, 1996

Stevenson J: Evidence for a genetic etiology in hyperactivity in children. Behav Genet 22:337–344, 1992

Stevenson J, Meares R: An outcome study of psychotherapy for patients with borderline personality disorder. Am J Psychiatry 149:358–362, 1992

Still GF: Some abnormal psychical conditions in children. Lancet 1:1108–1112, 1902

Stone L: The widening scope of indications for psychoanalysis. J Am Psychoanal Assoc 2:567–594, 1954

Stone MH: The Borderline Syndromes. New York, McGraw-Hill, 1980

Stone MH: Abnormalities of Personality. New York, Norton, 1993

Strauss J: Person–environment interaction in schizophrenia. Br J Psychiatry 161 (suppl 18):19–26, 1992

Strupp HH, Hadley SW: Specific vs. non-specific factors in psychotherapy. Arch Gen Psychiatry 36:1125–1136, 1979

Stunkard AJ, Sorenson TI, Hanics C: An adoption study of human obesity. N Engl J Med 314:193–198, 1986

Sullivan HS: The Interpersonal Theory of Psychiatry. New York, WW Norton, 1953

Sulloway F: Freud: Biologist of the Mind. New York, Basic Books, 1979

Sulloway F: Born to Rebel. New York, Pantheon, 1996

Summers KM: Genetic susceptibility to common diseases. Med J Aust 158:783–788, 1993

Tambs K, Sundet JM, Eaves L, et al: Genetic and environmental effects on type A scores in monozygotic twin families. Behav Genet 22:499–513, 1992

Tarter RE, Moss HB, Vanyukov MM: Behavioral genetics and the etiology of alcoholism, in The Genetics of Alcoholism. Edited by Begleiter H, Kissin B. New York, Oxford University Press, 1995, pp 294–326

Tellegen A, Lykken DT, Bouchard TJ, et al: Personality similarity in twins reared apart and together. J Pers Soc Psychol 54:1031–1039, 1988

Tennant C: Parental loss in childhood to adult life. Arch Gen Psychiatry 45: 1045–1050, 1988

Terr LC: What happens to early memories of trauma? J Am Acad Child Adolesc Psychiatry 27:96–104, 1988

Terr LC: Childhood traumas: an outline and an overview. Am J Psychiatry 148:10–20, 1991

Thaker GK, Cassady S, Adami H: Eye movements in spectrum personality disorders: comparison of community subjects and relatives of schizophrenic patients. Am J Psychiatry 153:362–368, 1996

Thapar A, McGuffin P: A twin study of depressive symptoms in childhood. Br J Psychiatry 165:259–265, 1994

Thapar A, McGuffin P: Genetic influences on life events. Psychol Med 26: 813–830, 1996

Thompson RA, Connell JP, Bridges LJ: Temperament, emotion, and social interactive behavior in the strange situation. Child Dev 56:1106–1110, 1988

Tienari P, Wynne LC, Moring J, et al: The Finnish adoptive family study of schizophrenia: implications for family research. Br J Psychiatry 23 (suppl): 20–26, 1994

Tiger L: Men in Groups. New York, Random House, 1969

Tillman JG, Nash MR, Lerner PR: Does trauma cause dissociative pathology? in Dissociation: Clinical and Theoretical Perspectives. Edited by Lynn SJ, Rhue JW. New York, Guilford, 1994, pp 395–414

Tooby J, Cosmides L: The psychological foundations of culture, in The Adapted Mind: Evolutionary Psychology and the Generation of Culture. Edited by Barkow JH, Cosmides L, Tooby J. New York, Oxford University Press, 1992, pp 19–136

Torgersen S: The oral, obsessive and hysterical personality syndromes: a study of heredity and environmental factors by means of the twin method. Arch Gen Psychiatry 37:1272–1277, 1980

Torgersen S: Genetic factors in anxiety disorders. Arch Gen Psychiatry 40: 1085–1089, 1983

Torgersen S: Genetic and nosological aspects of schizotypal and borderline personality disorders: a twin study. Arch Gen Psychiatry 41:546–554, 1984

Torgersen S: The psychometric–genetic structure of DSM-III personality disorder diagnostic criteria. Presented to the International Society for the Study of Personality Disorders, Oslo, Norway, July 1991

Torgersen S: Personality disorders in our genes? Presentation to the Second European Congress on Personality Disorders, Milan, Italy, June 1996

Torgersen S, Onstad S, Skre I, et al: "True" schizotypal personality disorder: a study of co-twins and relatives of schizophrenic probands. Am J Psychiatry 150:1661–1667, 1993

Torrey EF: Freudian Fraud. New York, Harper Perennial, 1992

Torrey EF, Bowler AE, Taylor EH, et al: Schizophrenia and Manic-Depressive Disorder. New York, Basic Books, 1994

Treasure J, Holland AJ: Genetic factors in eating disorders, in Handbook of Eating Disorders: Theory, Treatment and Research. Edited by Szmukler G, Dare C, Treasure J. Chichester, UK, John Wiley, 1995, pp 65–81

Trimble M: Post-traumatic stress disorder: history of a concept, in Trauma and Its Wake. Edited by Figley C. New York, Brunner/Mazel, 1985, pp 5–14

True WR, Rice J, Eisen SA, et al: A twin study of genetic and environmental contributions to liability for post-traumatic stress symptoms. Arch Gen Psychiatry 50:257–264, 1993

Tsuang MT, Gilbertson MW, Faraone S: Genetics of negative and positive symptoms in schizophrenia, in Positive Versus Negative Symptoms in Schizophrenia. Edited by Maneras A, Tsuang MT, Andreasen NA. New York, Springer Verlag, 1991, pp 265–271

Tucker GJ: Putting DSM-IV in perspective. Am J Psychiatry 155:159–161, 1998

Tylor E: Researches Into the Early History of Mankind (1895). Chicago, IL, University of Chicago Press, 1964

Tyrer P: Personality Disorders. London, Wright, 1988

Vaillant GE: Adaptation to Life. Cambridge, MA, Little, Brown, 1977

Vaillant GE: The Natural History of Alcoholism, 2nd Edition. Cambridge, MA, Harvard University Press, 1994

Vaillant GE: A long-term follow-up of male alcohol abuse. Arch Gen Psychiatry 53:243–249, 1996

Vaillant GE, Gerber PD: Natural history of male psychological health, XIII: who develops high blood pressure and who responds to treatment. Am J Psychiatry 153 (suppl):24–29, 1996

Valenstein ES: Great and Desperate Cures: The Rise and Decline of Psycho-surgery and Other Radical Treatments for Mental Illness. New York, Basic Books, 1986

Vandenberg SG, Singer SM, Pauls DL: The Heredity of Behavior Disorders in Adults and Children. New York, Plenum, 1986

van der Kolk BA: The body keeps the score: memory and the evolving psycho-biology of posttraumatic stress. Harv Rev Psychiatry 1:253–265, 1994

van der Kolk BA, Perry JC, Herman JL: Childhood origins of self-destructive behavior. Am J Psychiatry 148:1665–1671, 1991

Vanderveycken W, van Deth R: From Fasting Saints to Anorexic Girls: The History of Self-Starvation. New York, New York University Press, 1994

Vitousek K, Manke F: Personality variables and disorders in anorexia nervosa and bulimia nervosa. J Abnorm Psychol 103:137–147, 1994

Wachtel PL: Psychoanalysis and Behavior Therapy. New York, Basic Books, 1977

Wachtel PL: Therapeutic Communication. New York, Guilford, 1993

Wachtel PL: Cyclical processes in personality and psychopathology. J Abnorm Psychol 103:51–54, 1994

Wahlberg KE, Wynne LC, Oja H, et al: Gene-environment interaction in vulnerability to schizophrenia: findings from the Finnish adoptive family study of schizophrenia. Am J Psychiatry 154:355–362, 1997

Wallerstein J: Second Chances: Men, Women, and Children a Decade After Divorce. New York, Ticknor & Fields, 1989

Wallerstein R: Forty-Two Lives in Treatment. New York, Guilford, 1986

Watson J: Behaviorism (1926). New York, Norton, 1970

Webster S: Why Freud Was Wrong. New York, Basic Books, 1995

Weinberg RA: How cancers arise. Sci Am 275:62–70, 1996

Weinberger DR: Implications of normal brain development for the pathogenesis of schizophrenia. Arch Gen Psychiatry 44:660–669, 1987

Weiner H: Psychobiology and Human Disease. New York, Brunner/Mazel, 1977

Weiss G, Hechtman L: Hyperactive Children Grown Up, 2nd Edition. New York, Guilford, 1992

Weiss M, Zelkowitz P, Feldman R, et al: Psychopathology in offspring of mothers with borderline personality disorder. Can J Psychiatry 41:285–290, 1996

Weissenbach J, Gyapy G, Dib C: A second generation linkage map of the human genome. Nature 359:794–801, 1992

Weissman MM: Family genetic studies of panic disorder. J Psychiatr Res 27 (suppl 1):69–78, 1993

Weissman MM, Klerman GL: Gender and depression. Trends Neurosci 8:416–420, 1985

Weissman MM, Leaf PJ, Tischler GL, et al: Affective disorders in five United States communities. Psychol Med 18:141–153, 1988

Weissman MM, Wickramaratne P, Adams PB: The relationship between panic disorder and depression. Arch Gen Psychiatry 50:767–780, 1993

Weissman MM, Bland RC, Canino GJ, et al: Cross-national epidemiology of major depressive and bipolar disorder. JAMA 276:298–299, 1996

Wender PH: The Hyperactive Child, Adolescent, and Adult: Attention Deficit Disorder Through the Lifespan. New York, Oxford University Press, 1987

Werner EE, Smith RS: Overcoming the Odds: High Risk Children From Birth to Adulthood. New York, Cornell University Press, 1992

Wessley S: Mental illness as metaphor, yet again. BMJ 314:153, 1997

Westermeyer J: Historical and social context of psychoactive substance disorders, in Clinical Textbook of Addictive Disorders. Edited by Frances RJ, Miller SI. New York, Guilford, 1991, pp 23–42

Wiborg IM, Dahl AA: Does brief dynamic psychotherapy reduce the relapse rate of panic disorder? Arch Gen Psychiatry 53:689–694, 1996

Williams GH: Hypertension, in Harrison's Principles of Internal Medicine, 12th Edition. Edited by Braunwald F, Isselbacher KJ, Wilson JD, et al. New York, McGraw-Hill, 1994, pp 1116–1131

Williams RB, Barefoot JC, Califf RM: Prognostic importance of social and economic resources among medically treated patients with angiographically documented coronary artery disease. JAMA 267:520–524, 1992

Williams RR: Nature, nurture, and family predisposition. N Engl J Med 318:769–771, 1988

Wilson EO: Sociobiology: The New Synthesis. Cambridge, MA, Harvard University Press, 1975

Winnicott DW: Collected Papers. London, Tavistock, 1958

Winokur G, Clayton PJ, Reich T: Manic-Depressive Illness. St Louis, MO, CV Mosby, 1969

Wise MG, Gray KF: Delirium, dementia, and amnestic disorders, in The American Psychiatric Press Textbook of Psychiatry, 2nd Edition. Edited by Hales RE, Yudofsky SC, Talbott JA. Washington, DC, American Psychiatric Press, 1994, pp 311–354

Wolf ME, Mosnaim AD (eds): Posttraumatic Stress Disorder: Etiology, Phenomenology, and Treatment. Washington, DC, American Psychiatric Press, 1990

World Health Organization: Schizophrenia: An International Pilot Study. New York, Wiley, 1979

World Health Organization: International Classification of Diseases, 10th Edition. Geneva, Switzerland, World Health Organization, 1992

Wright R: The Moral Animal. New York, Pantheon, 1994

Wyatt RJ: Neuroleptics and the natural course of schizophrenia. Schizophr Bull 17:325–351, 1991

Wyshak G: The relation between change in reports of traumatic events and symptoms of psychiatric distress. Gen Hosp Psychiatry 16:290–297, 1994

Yehuda R, McFarlane AC: Conflict between current knowledge about posttraumatic stress disorder and its original conceptual basis. Am J Psychiatry 152:1705–1713, 1995

Yehuda R, Elkin A, Binder-Byrnes K, et al: Dissociation in aging Holocaust survivors. Am J Psychiatry 153:935–940, 1996

Yochelson S, Samenow S: The Criminal Personality. New York, Jason Aronson, 1976

Young A: Harmony of Illusions. Princeton, NJ, Princeton University Press, 1995

Zeitlin D: The Natural History of Psychiatric Disorders in Children. Oxford, UK, Oxford University Press, 1986

Zoccolillo M: Co-occurrence of conduct disorder and its adult outcomes with depressive and anxiety disorders: a review. J Am Acad Child Adolesc Psychiatry 32:547–556, 1992

Zoccolillo M, Pickles A, Quinton D, et al: The outcome of childhood conduct disorder: implications for defining adult personality disorder and conduct disorder. Psychol Med 22:971–986, 1992

Zubin J, Steinhauer SR, Condray R: Vulnerability to relapse in schizophrenia. Br J Psychiatry 18 (suppl):13–18, 1992

Zweig-Frank H, Paris J, Guzder J: Psychological risk factors for dissociation and self-mutilation in female patients with personality disorders. Can J Psychiatry 39:259–265, 1994a

Zweig-Frank H, Paris J, Guzder J: Psychological risk factors for self-mutilation in male patients with personality disorders. Can J Psychiatry 39:266–268, 1994b

Zweig-Frank H, Paris J, Guzder J: Psychological risk factors for dissociation in female patients with borderline and non-borderline personality disorders. J Personal Disord 8:203–209, 1994c

Zweig-Frank H, Paris J, Guzder J: Dissociation in male patients with borderline and non-borderline personality disorders. J Personal Disord 8:210–218, 1994d

Index

Page numbers printed in **boldface** *type refer to tables or figures.*